STAYING HEALTHY

HEALTHY

—IN—

MODERN

INDIA

PRACTICAL ADVICE FOR LIVING A HEALTHY LIFE AND TACKLING DISEASE

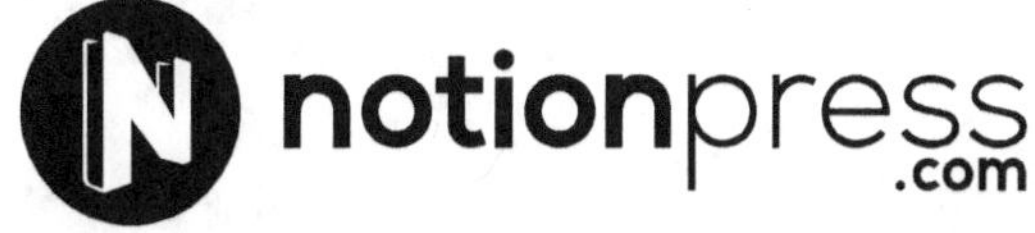

STAYING HEALTHY
IN
MODERN INDIA

PRACTICAL ADVICE FOR LIVING A
HEALTHY LIFE AND TACKLING DISEASE

Dr. Gita Mathai, MBBS, DCH

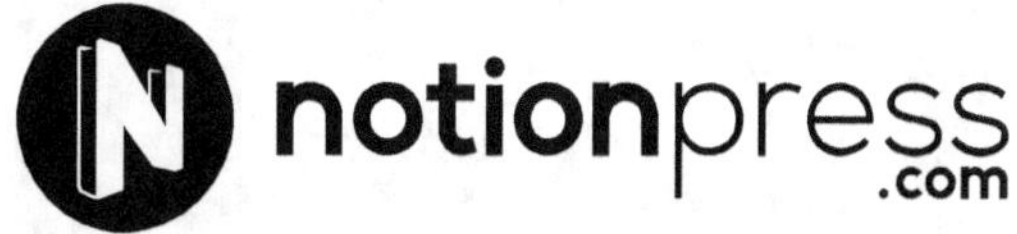

Notion Press

Old No. 38, New No. 6
McNichols Road, Chetpet
Chennai - 600 031

First Published by Notion Press 2016
Copyright © Dr. Gita Mathai 2016
All Rights Reserved.

ISBN 978-93-86009-93-7

This book is dedicated to

My Alma Mater

Christian Medical College Vellore

And the dedicated teachers who inspired all who were
fortunate enough to study there.

After being in family practice for over three decades, in semi-rural India, and visiting many other countries like the USA, UK, Thailand, Singapore and Korea, I discovered that when it comes to approaching physicians, race and ethnicity are irrelevant. People all over the world are the same. They set about seeking a physician with hesitation and trepidation, fearful of the diagnosis and outcome of the disease.

Quite often, in a world filled with specialists and super specialists, they are not sure of whom to consult and where to turn. Things can go haywire when the person goes to the wrong department or super specialty. They often end up doing expensive and sometimes irrelevant tests. A great deal of time lapses before they find their way back to the appropriate department – and finally receive a diagnosis.

I started writing health columns more than 15 years ago. I received substantial feedback from my readers. There were many many queries which inundated my inbox. Soon, I realized that health, exercise and weight loss and aging are foremost on people's minds. People want answers. They want to know why they were ill, (is it an act of God? Is it genetic?) how they could tackle it at home till they got an appointment, and which specialist they should consult.

I hope that by compiling these articles, the book will address these issues, clear doubts and provide easy practical solutions to simple problems.

This book is dedicated

My husband Dr. Dilip Mathai

My parents Dr. Easo John and late Leelamani John

My children Kamini and Anith,

Son in law Philip, daughter-in law Dr. Lindsey Knake

And grandson Adiv

CONTENTS

About the Book

Everyone in the family seems to be writing books. My father wrote two in the space of one year on management. My daughter, between pregnancy, delivery and weaning has written a biography of AR Rehmaan. My husband wrote a guide to the rational treatment of infectious diseases, Not to be out done, and demanding my fair share of computer time, I decided to compile a collection of articles, my practical approach to health and wellbeing.

These articles were a pleasure to write and I hope that anyone who reads this book will find some useful tips.

ACKNOWLEDGEMENTS AND THANKS TO

The Telegraph Kolkotta

The New Indian Express,

Dr. Easo John for editorial help,

Dr. Leslie Margolin Professor of Creative Writing University of Iowa USA for guidance and teaching me to write.

CHAPTER 1

MEDICAL CONSULTATIONS— AND WHAT THEY MEAN

Why? When? What?

Visiting a doctor professionally causes anxiety, and patients are happy to find reasons to avoid the inevitable. Once the decision has been made to seek expert advice, either to have a health check up or to evaluate a serious symptom, it is better to take the first step and go to a physician as soon as possible. Women tend to do this initially, but then are less likely to follow through with the recommendations. Men more likely to seek a face saving escape route and refuse to go.

It is not only disease and disability that require medical consultations. There are a multitude of advantageous preventive services available, to maintain health, which with increased public awareness, can be effectively utilized.

The emphases during a health check up in the different age groups vary. Children need an evaluation every month during the first year and twice a year subsequently. The growth (height weight) teeth, eyes, ears and skin need to be checked. Adolescents, ready to go to college, need advice about the dangers of drugs, alcohol, smoking and sex.

The immunization requirements in the various age groups are also different. Children should follow the IAP (Indian association of paediatrics) immunization schedule. All the recommended immunizations are not provided free by the government. The schedule also gets modified periodically. New medical advances and research mean that immunizations may be added to an existing schedule.

Have your paediatrician check your immunization record periodically. It is not just children who need to be immunized. Some immunizations are required even in adult life. College going children should have their DT, hepatitis B hepatitis A, and typhoid boosters before leaving home. (A detailed schedule is available in the next chapter).

Men and women need evaluation of weight, blood pressure, blood sugars, cholesterol and lipids. Based on the results, further follow up may be needed. Advice regarding adherence to an appropriate diet, and getting sufficient exercise, is needed for all ages and both sexes, especially with our increasingly sedentary unhealthy urban life style.

At certain stages like menarche, marriage, pregnancy, lactation and menopause, women need specialized care and advice. In addition they need a "pap smear" for cancer every three years until the age of 65. Some physicians also recommend a mammogram after the age of 45 every 2–3 years.

When visiting a doctor, you should have a clear idea of your requirements.

Everyone carries their individualized baggage of anxieties; apprehensions and queries. A written checklist of all the questions you want answered saves time, especially as the stress of the consultation may cause a memory lapse and leave unexplained unexpressed queries.

It is better to fix an appointment and then arrive a few minutes early, rather than to breathlessly rush in at the last minute requesting an "adjustment" into the doctor's already tight schedule.

Take all old medical documents, investigations, radiographs and prescriptions along.

The doctor may have some questions and it is better to be prepared with the answers.

"Is this a routine check up or do you have any symptoms?"

"Do you have a family history of medical conditions like allergies, diabetes, hypertension, heart attacks or infectious diseases such as tuberculosis?"

"Is there a recent change in your weight?"

"Do you smoke drink or use drugs?"

You should be prepared with accurate background information including pregnancies, abortions, immunizations and previous illnesses.

Sensitive topics, especially those dealing with sex may cause embarrassment, be related to the back of the mind or avoided all together. This is self-defeating, as you will finish the consultation and leave with unresolved doubts. Written questions can be read out and answered without embarrassing eye contact.

After completing medical college and practicing for a few years, there is very little a doctor has not heard or seen.

Having a friend or relative present helps with precise recall of the professional communication if confidentiality is not an issue. On the other hand this may be self- defeating as you may not be able to express all your questions or fears.

A physical examination is usually part of the evaluation process, so wear clothes that can be removed and put on again without much difficulty.

Once the consultation is over, there are some questions that you may like to ask so that there is no miscommunication.

"Are these tests really needed?"

"What is the diagnosis? What does it mean? Does it affect my family? Do I need to evaluate any of them for a similar or related problem?"

"Is there any way, with diet, exercise or a change in life style, to reduce the number of medications taken?"

"How do I take these tablets? How many times a day and for how long? Are they taken before or after food? Are there any side defects?"

"How long do I have to wait for improvement?"

"Is this a disease (like diabetes or hypertension) where I will require lifelong evaluation and treatment?"

"When do I need to return for follow up?"

For your own safety, make sure all findings are permanently documented. Keep a personal file with your own record of illnesses and medicines.

If a surgical procedure has been advised, it is probably wiser to get a second opinion before proceeding with what may eventually be inevitable.

Check all prescription medications and make sure you understand what they are for, when they should be taken, and the number of doses per day and the total duration of the treatment. Ensure that they are the drugs the doctor has prescribed and not what the pharmacy has substituted. Check the expiry dates of medications. If in doubt, return to the physician for clarifications.

Misconstruction of medical communication is a common phenomenon.

"If I swallow these will I become thin?" asked the overweight woman, as she looked hopefully at the large bottle of brightly coloured tablets.

"No," replied the doctor, "that is not what I said".

"Then?"

" You are supposed to drop them on the floor, and pick them up on one a time, three times a day."

This scenario is not as bizarre as it sounds. There is often a failure of lucid communication between the people involved during medical consultations, with the busy physician and apprehensive patient talking at cross-purposes. In short, there is a discrepancy between what is said and what is heard. We hear what we want to hear. This why personal documentation and a personal file are important.

With a little care, attention to detail and documentation of facts, medical consultations can be pleasurable, beneficial and stress free.

CHAPTER 2

IMMUNIZATIONS

"Preventive Pokes" Are our children pincushions?

Gone are the days when childhood immunization consisted of a painful punch injection of small pox vaccine followed three months later by the intramuscular administration of "triple antigen" and polio drops. Immunization is now a big business as more and more diseases can be prevented by injections.

As a country we have a good track record as far as immunization is concerned. The government health services provide BCG , 3 doses of DPT (triple antigen) and OPV(oral polio vaccine) or IPV (Injectable Polio Vaccine) and measles vaccine free of cost. Boosters are administered at the ages of one and a half years and five years.

The government has done a good job. The greater part of the population is covered. Essential immunization (not ideal) is also provided free of cost at primary health centres and in the government hospitals to children who go there to the age of five years. The IAP (Indian Association of Paediatrics) has recommended a schedule which extends up to 16 years.

Trained paramedical personnel also pay home visits to weigh children and administer vaccines. In some states like Tamil Nadu, the health workers do their job efficiently, moving from house to house, immunizing children and pregnant women, creating health awareness, advising spacing and contraception, weighing children and keeping tabs on weaning and nutrition. In some other states the situation is not as satisfactory.

Growth charts with comprehensive immunization schedules printed at the back are commercially available from infant food manufacturers and many private organizations. Despite all this, there are misconceptions, myths and misinformation about which immunizations should be taken, when they should be administered, where the vaccines are available, possible side effects and relative contraindications.

Unfortunately, we still have an infant mortality rate of 64 per 1000 children, which is higher than that in several other developing countries with a per capita income less than ours. Many of these children die due to infectious diseases. Some infections are due to an unsanitary environment, with unclean water and unhygienic sewage disposal facilities. Others are preventable, with proper immunization.

Some extra vaccines are recommended as part of an extended immunization schedule. Unfortunately, the availability and necessity of these vaccinations is not publicized. Public awareness is minimal. The injections are not subsidized or free.

This arouses queries arise in the minds of parents:

- ➤ Are these immunizations are really necessary?
- ➤ If so, why are they not offered by the government?
- ➤ Why are they not a part of the national immunization program?

Silence on the part of the government, and inertia in countering negative publicity about extra immunizations can have disastrous effects on the health of our country.

Parents are expected to purchase "optional" vaccine for administration to their children. Many private clinics and hospitals offer them as an "extended" immunization schedule. Some are expensive, but they are all needed.

From birth to the age of 16 years, the following is the general schedule followed:

- ➤ Birth BCG, Hep B, OPV
- ➤ 6weeks (1 ½ months) DPT, OPV, Hep B, Hib, pneumococcal vaccine
- ➤ 10 weeks (2 ½ months) DPT, OPV, Hib pneumococcal vaccine

- ➤ 14 weeks (3 ½ months) DPT, OPV Hep B, Hib pneumococcal vaccine
- ➤ Rotavirus 2 injections
- ➤ 10 months Measles
- ➤ After 1 year Varicella vaccine (chicken pox)
- ➤ 15 month (1 year and 3 months) MMR
- ➤ 18 months (1 ½ years) DPT, OPV /pneumococcal vaccine booster
- ➤ 2 years Typhoid vaccine, Hep A (2 doses 4 to 6 months apart)
- ➤ 5 yrs DPT, OPV, Hep B booster
- ➤ Human papillovirus between 9–11 years 3 doses 0,1,6
- ➤ 10 yrs dT/OPV /MMR
- ➤ 16 yrs dT/OPV

BCG (Bacille Calmette Guerin. Initially publicized as a preventive measure for tuberculosis it is offered free by the government. There has been some controversy about it in recent times. The general consensus is that it does offer a measure of protection against tuberculous meningitis, which is the most dangerous and fatal form of tuberculosis.

OPV (Oral polio vaccine). It can be replaced with IPV. It protects against paralytic polio and is provided free.

The government also conducts camps which are publicized. The vaccine is administered in pulses on a single day to all the children to boost the immunity of the entire country and to reduce spread of the wild polio virus.

DPT This is "triple antigen" which offers protection against diphtheria, tetanus and whooping cough. It is offered free by the government.

dT (dual antigen) is given after the age of 5 years instead of DPT. It contains a smaller dose of diphtheria and the usual dose tetanus. It is also preferred over the traditional DPT before Hib age of 5 if the child has a seizure disorder. It is not given free by the government. The government program stops at the age of 5 years.

Hep B (Hepatitis B). The government does not issue this free. However NGOs offer vaccination at lower costs in regular camps. Three doses have to be given, at 0–30days and 6 months. It then provides life long immunity. Sometimes the organizers of the camp do not turn up to administer the third dose. If such is the case it can be bought at a pharmacy and administered by a medical person. Also the correct dose (0.5ml in children and 1 ml in adults) has to be given on the muscular upper 1/3 of the arm or the thigh. It should not be given in the fat laden buttocks.

If an unimmunized person develops a preventable disease like hepatitis B, recovery may be complete with no sequalae. The disease can be fatal in 1%, or may progress to a carrier state, chronic hepatitis or liver cancer. A mother who is a carrier for hepatitis B may have her condition detected accidentally by blood tests done during pregnancy. If such is the case the newborn child should have immunoglobulin administered at birth. Also the husband's status needs to be checked. If he is negative he needs to be immunized as one of the methods of spread of the disease is through sex.

If immunizations are missed before the age of 1 year it can be taken at any age at intervals of 0, 1, 6 months.

Hib This offers protection against brain fever (meningitis) due to H Influenzae type b. If the immunization has been missed before the age of 1 year a single dose can be administered between the ages of one and two. It is not advised after the age of two. It is not given free by the government. The cases of meningitis have fallen drastically in areas where active propaganda and immunization are being carried on.

MMR protects against measles, mumps and rubella (German measles). Although by itself Rubella is a mild illness, if acquired during pregnancy it causes the dreaded "congenital rubella syndrome" producing an abnormal baby with a small head, deafness, heart disease, cataract in both eyes and many other problems. Boosters are advised in some countries at the age of five and again at ten. It is not free.

Rubella vaccine alone is available for administration as a single injection for unimmunized adolescents who have already had mumps and measles. Unimmunized women planning marriage should be immunized at least a month before the date of the wedding. Women embarking on fertility interventions should definitely review their immune status and complete the schedule before treatment is started.

Typhoid vaccine is available commercially in two forms. There are oral capsules to be swallowed on an empty stomach on days 1, 3 and 5 or the simpler single injection. It produces hardly any reaction and is not the older TAB vaccine, which though cheaper had many side effects like pain and fever. TAB vaccine also produced less immunity. The cost of the oral form and the injection is almost the same. It is not free. The immunization has to be repeated every 3 years.

Hep A The injection for hepatitis A administered as two injections 4 to 6 months apart. No boosters are required as it provides life long immunity. It is not free.

Varicella Vaccine is given to prevent chicken pox. No boosters are required. It is not free.

dT boosters have to be taken every 10 years.

If schedules are not correctly followed, and boosters missed, you are likely to get the infections. Some immunizations are now combined commercially so that the number of pokes is reduced.

Newer vaccines are against pneumoccus, human papillovirus and rotavirus

Live vaccines should not be given to immuno-compromised individuals. Please check with your health care provider.

Currently there is no commercially available vaccine for AIDS or malaria. Research is on going and a breakthrough may occur any day.

All countries require a tourist to take certain immunizations before travel. They are usually listed in the visa application form. Allow at least a month for completing the required immunization.

During epidemics the government provided extra immunizations. Some, like the injections offered for cholera are only 40% effective.

Influenza vaccine against "flu" does not offer protection across the board but is specific for that particular strain of virus.

Optional immunizations, as the following are labelled, are recommended by the WHO (world health organization) and by the IAP (Indian association of Paediatrics). They are MMR Vaccine (Measles mumps and rubella), Chicken pox vaccine, Typhoid (oral or injection), Hepatitis B, Hepatitis A and Hib (H Influenzae meningitis).

Meninigococcal, pneumococcal and influenza vaccines are recommended for particular groups of children and adults. Rabies vaccine should be administered in all cases of cat, dog, cow, horse or monkey bite.

Although some of these infections like mumps and chicken pox appear innocuous , in 10% of the children there can be devastating permanent damage to the internal organs and brain. Typhoid is easily treatable, but infection causes loss of school days. Rubella (German measles) if acquired during pregnancy can cause abnormal babies. Hepatitis B infection can lead to a carrier state and liver cancer.

Japanese B encephalitis causes a particular brain fever that has nothing to do with Japan, and it has aroused very little publicity or government interest. Yet, children are already dead, and more people are getting infected every day. Some survive, but they are not the lucky ones. They are left with permanent devastating sequelae like paralysis, seizures, blindness, deafness and mental retardation.

This infection is caused by a virus. It is transmitted by the Culex mosquito which acquires it from an amplification reservoir of infected pigs and wild fowl. It is not transmitted person-to- person.

Once infected, there is no cure with miracle drugs or antibiotics. Affected children have to "ride out" the disease with supportive treatment.

This disease is a tragedy, as it is entirely preventable with adequate and timely immunization.

India manufactures vaccines against Japanese B encephalitis both in the public and private sector. The recommended dosage schedule is in the package insert, and is usually 0,7,30 days for children above the age of one. The immunity conferred is between 93–97%. Now, China has manufactured and released a new cheaper vaccine which can be administered as a single injection. Despite the epidemic, little publicity has been given to promoting the vaccine.

Schools can help to create immunization awareness by asking parents to submit a copy of the immunizations administered to the child at the time of admission; along with the birth certificate and other documents. By making sure that all the children in the school are protected against vaccine preventable diseases, the number of school days lost by the children as a result of infections will be significantly reduced.

We are now trying as a nation to promote the small family norm. We have moved from "we two ours two" to "we two ours one".

This gives us a sacred duty to keep our children's immunization schedules up to date.

So, if you have them, immunize them!

Chapter 3

Tackling Fever

Man is a warm-blooded mammal. To remain comfortable, our internal temperature must be maintained within normal limits by a natural thermostat in the part called the hypothalamus in our brain. This switches itself on and off as it adjusts the temperature, based on signals received from the peripheral nerves. It functions like the thermostat in the refrigerator or air-conditioner. Temperature has a normal circadian rhythm. It is maximum between 4 and 8 pm and lowest between 2 am and 6 am.

Fever is neither a subjective feeling nor a disease entity. It is a symptom that can be measured and demonstrated to be above the normal value of 98.6 degrees Fahrenheit by thermometers. It is caused by a rise in the core temperature in response to heat producing particles called pyrogens released by invading bacteria, viruses, or tumour producing cells, or as a response to autoimmune disease. Fever is not harmful. It is the body's efficient defence mechanism against disease.

If the internal temperature rises, sweating mechanisms come into play, which cause evaporation of water from the skin and a reduction in the temperature. A drop in the outside temperature causes shivering, which increases muscle activity and elevates the internal core temperature. Accompanying constriction of the peripheral blood vessels reduces heat loss by conduction and convection.

Parents feel helpless and do not know how to tackle the fever in their children. They fear that a rise in temperature will cause brain damage and seizures. This results in "fever phobia" with inappropriate responses from parents and caregivers.

Other parents are anxious and feel that the child is unhealthy and "always sick." A normal healthy child has a steady weight gain. However there may be 6 to 8 febrile episodes a year in the first two years of life. If each fever lasts for 7 days, this means that the normal child has been ill for 40 days a year. Recurrent fever is a child is defined as 3 or more febrile episodes in a 6-month period occurring at least 7 days apart with no obvious causative medical illness. Continuous fever, is fever present every day for 14 days.

In 80 % of the children, fever is viral and will settle down in three to five days time. In 20 % it is a manifestation of a serious infection. Doctors have to balance" masterly inactivity and a "wait and watch" approach with timely investigation and intervention.

Some children develop "febrile" seizures at the height of the fever. There are usually no neurological signs and there may be a family history of similar episodes. In such children the slightest suspicion of fever warrants first aid measures. The temperature should be reduced with tepid sponging and paracetemol before consulting the doctor.

A physician must be consulted,

➢ If the infant is less than a month old

➢ Seems too ill to drink fluids adequately

➢ Is dehydrated

➢ Has seizures

➢ Is still febrile after 72 hours

➢ Has inconsolable crying and irritability

➢ Is confused or delirious

➢ Has rash

➢ There is difficulty in breathing

➢ To reduce the fever adequate doses of anti pyretic medication must be given at the correct intervals. The decision to start should be based on "touch, " a feeling of "heat" or "exhaustion." The temperature should be recorded using a "digital thermometer." It can be placed in the armpit or under the tongue. As soon as the body temperature is recorded it "bleeps." Medication should be given only if the temperature is more than 100.5 F.

The dosage is not dependent on the age but the weight. Paracetemol should be given in the strength of 10–15 mg /kg per dose every 4–6 hours. The paediatric tablets contain 125 mg, the syrups contain 125 mg (usually in 5ml or 1 teaspoon.) Ibubrufen suspension can be used instead of paracetemol every 6 hours in the same dose. Aspirin is not safe in children under the age of 10 years unless specifically prescribed for certain fevers by the doctor. It can precipitate the dreaded Reyes syndrome with renal and brain involvement in certain viral infections. This can be fatal in 50 % of the cases.

Dehydration due to inadequate fluid intake causes fever to rise. Hence adequate hydration should be maintained.

In addition to the above measures, dress the child in light clothes. Warm clothing and "bundling" causes the temperature to rise in children, as their sweating mechanism is still relatively immature. Wipe the unclothed body with a towel soaked in water at room temperature and allow the water to evaporate under a fan. Do not use warm water or soak the child in ice water.

Before going to the doctor check

- If the child has a rash

- Is constantly rubbing a ear (earache)

- Has any painful red cuts or bruises

- Has abdominal pain

- Has any swellings

When you do consult a doctor, be sure to carry your immunization records with you. The government provides free immunization against diseases like diphtheria, whooping cough tetanus, polio and measles and boosters up to the age of five years. Other immunizations have to be purchased and are not provided free in primary health centres and government hospitals. Brain fever (HiB), chicken pox, MMR (measles mumps and rubella) typhoid and hepatitis A are preventable diseases which cause fever. These diseases can be automatically eliminated in the differential diagnosis if the immunization schedule is complete.

Remember, if immunization has been timely and adequate with appropriate boosters many infections can be automatically ruled out. This helps in speed and accuracy of diagnosis and makes the doctor's job easier. It is better to immunize in time and be safe rather than be sorry later.

Consult a physician if your child is sick, but follow first aid measures first. Reduce the temperature to the best of your ability at home. When you visit the doctor, insist on documentation of all injections and generic medications administered. Maintain a file for each child so there is no ambiguity, and a rational decision can be made about treatment or further evaluation.

Any fever that persists for more than five days needs medical evaluation. Remember, fever is a symptom of many diseases. All fevers are not the same. It is the body's natural safety device against disease.

Chapter 4

Solutions for Diarrhoea

- ➤ 1 level teaspoon of salt.
- ➤ 8 level teaspoons of sugar;
- ➤ 1000 ml of boiled cooled water

Taste the solution you have just made. It should not be more salty than tears. This is the basic homemade ORS (Oral Rehydration Solution), recommended by the World Health Organization, which has revolutionalized the treatment of diarrhoea all over the world. A lifesaving solution cannot be cheaper!

This solution keeps the person hydrated and reduces the mortality caused by diarrhoea. It does not however tackle the agent causing the disease or reduce the total duration of the illness. This can be frustrating as there is no apparent decrease in the frequency and quantity of the stool.

ORS (for rehydration) is sold in pharmacies as readymade powder sachets or as the more expensive bottled 'ready-to-drink' solutions. ORS sachets when purchased should be reconstituted in the RECOMMENDED amount of previously measured boiled cooled water. If the water is too little it will increase the concentration of the ORS and may cause hypernatraemia (high sodium content), which is dangerous in the young and elderly. If the solution is too dilute, it is not every effective. Water should be boiled and cooled before being added to the ORS powder. Boiling ORS after it is prepared alters the electrolyte constitution and caramelizes the sugar making it useless. If vomiting accompanies the diarrhoea, feeding small quantities of the solution at frequent intervals helps. ORS does not reduce the frequency of the stools, it only PREVENTS dehydration. This is often distressing to the affected individual who feels that they are not getting better.

The palatability of the ORS can be increased, and the frequency of diarrhoea reduced if starches like rice are added. Ready to use rice based ORS sachets are marketed. Alternatively, equal quantities of rice and dal can be cooked at home in a pressure cooker, mashed well and salt added to taste. It should then be boiled once more with additional water to make it the consistency of gruel (Kanji).

Mashed bananas are easily digested and well tolerated during a diarrhoeal episode. They help with correction of electrolytes lost during the diarrhoea.

Fruit juices, fermented foods, and sweet colas and carbonated drinks should be avoided.

Most acute diarrhoea subside on their own, and recovery is spontaneous provided hydration is maintained.

All diarrhoeas do not have a common cause, and therefore there is no 'universal' magic bullet to treat diarrhoea.

Diarrhoea may be sparked off by a food allergy, food poisoning, infection with bacteria or virus or infestation with parasites.

Food poisoning has an explosive onset 2 to 34 hours after ingestion of contaminated food. Usually, more than one person is affected, though the severity may vary from person to person. There is spontaneous recovery in 48 hours.

Diarrhoea caused by food allergies (seafood, nuts etc) is usually recognized by the patient or parent, is usually self limiting, and recurs with each dietary indiscretion.

Viral diarrhoeas are watery, there is little or no fever, and with adequate rehydration, recovery occurs spontaneously in 48 hours.

Sometimes people dose themselves with entroquinols (Mexaform Enteroquin) purchased OTC (over the counter) from the pharmacies. These are banned drugs. They cross the blood brain barrier especially in children. They are contraindicated in children.

Others take single self administered doses of the quinolones (the lox family-ciploxoflox, gatiflox) or trimethoprim combinations (Septran) or metronidazole (Flagyl, Metrogyl). They do not really "cure" diarrhoea, in this dose. They only suppress it and then contribute to the emergence of resistant organisms. These antibiotics should be taken in adequate prescribed doses for the correct duration. Only then are they effective. Lomotil and Lomofen suppress diarrhoea by reducing gastric emptying time and slowing intestinal motility. They can cause abdominal bloating and are dangerous in children and the elderly.

A doctor should be consulted in cases of diarrhoea if urine has not been passed for six hours, if there is high fever, intractable vomiting, alteration in the consciousness, severe cramping abdominal pain or if the diarrhoea has persisted for more than 48 hours.

Chronic diarrhoea persisting for more than 14 days needs expert evaluation.

A few simple precautions can be taken in summer to prevent diarrhoea.

Do not buy food which has been exposed to flies, sold in the open or touched by an ungloved food handler. If you are drinking fresh juice, the cleanliness of the food processor, and the source of the ice cubes should be checked.

Diarrhoea often occurs during holidays. Holidays are meant to expand our mental horizons, reduce stress and help us to cope with the demands of a challenging and changing world. They are meant to be enjoyed, with value for the money spent. None of these aims can be achieved if the entire focus of the trip shifts to the distance and availability of the nearest toilet.

Travel exposes friendly commensal bacteria living in our intestines to sudden changes in temperature and nutrition. Suddenly, they cease to be benevolent. Some of them are attacked and defeated by disease producing alien viruses, parasites or bacteria. Others mutate and mingle with the enemy forces. The body is simply no longer able to cope with the onslaught. The result is nausea, bloating, vomiting and diarrhoea, alone or in various uncomfortable combinations.

By following several simple guidelines while travelling, it is possible to avoid this embarrassing and distressing situation.

- ➢ Avoid raw foods. Fruits presented cut and peeled and may look attractive, but they can be contaminated with organisms. Fresh salads can tempt the calorie conscious, but their hygiene is open to question.

- ➢ Partially cooked or grilled "medium rare" meats can be a hotbed of disease producing bacteria.

- ➢ Sea fish, especially if stored in less than ideal conditions, may be "spoilt" and contain biotoxins. These can produce profuse watery diarrhoea, and sometimes tingling of the nerves and muscle weakness. Some have a high level of histidine which can be converted by the human body into the allergy rash producing histamine.

- ➢ Unpasteurized milk and milk products such as cheese provide a fertile medium for diarrhoea producing toxin releasing bacteria to grow.

- ➢ Food eaten from the roadside may suit the budget but not the palate. It is often unhygienic or served in inadequately washed unclean containers. It should be eaten only if it is piping hot.

- ➢ Only mineral or bottled water or hot tea or coffee should be drunk. If this is unavailable, water is safe after being boiled for a full minute. Or, alternatively, 5 drops (0.3 ml) of a 2% solution of tincture of iodine can be added to a litre of water. It should then be allowed to stand for 30 minutes before it is consumed.

- ➢ The outside of the bottle can or cup may be dirty and contaminated. Water can be directly drunk from the bottle by pouring it into the mouth from a distance. Otherwise, wipe any suspicious or unclean surface with which the mouth may have contact.

- ➢ If there is water borne epidemic like cholera in the destination, even the water used to brush the teeth can cause the disease. It is better to use "safe water" for everything other than bathing.

- ➢ Airline food is not necessarily safe. It may have been ordered at competitive rates from unhygienic local caterers.

Once the inevitable has occurred the most important measure is to remain hydrated. Roughly estimate the fluid loss with the diarrhoea and vomiting. This can be evaluated by monitoring the urine output and ensuring that the urine is not concentrated or high coloured. Drink enough fluids to replace this loss. Remember thirst is a sign of dehydration.

Fluids that can be safely used are

➤ Weak black tea with a little sugar

➤ Plain soda

➤ Commercially available ORS sachets. These are now available all over the world. They should be reconstituted carefully as directed to maintain the electrolyte balance.

➤ Home made ORS can be made with 6 teaspoons of sugar and ½ tsp of salt in a liter of water

➤ Rice gruel (conjee) made with double cooked rice and adequate salt.

Sometimes the excitement of travel, the change in the climate and the difference in the time zones can produce a temporary malfunction of the intestines. There may be a self limited increase in the frequency of the stools. This usually subsides spontaneously in a day. Before becoming unduly worried about the diarrhoea, hydrate yourself adequately and wait and watch for 24 hours.

Dysentery is differentiated from diarrhoea by the fact that it produces fever and diarrhoea with blood and mucous in the stool. It will usually respond to a 3–5 day course of ciprofloxacin 500 mg taken twice a day. Ciprofloxacin cannot be given to children or pregnant women.

Giardiasis causes bloating, stomach cramps, nausea, frequent gas and watery, foul-smelling diarrhoea. Amoebiasis has a more gradual in the onset, with cramping abdominal pain and blood and mucous in the stool. Both can appear several weeks after the initial exposure and persist until treated. Amoebiasis also can cause other health problems. Treatment for both is with a single 2 gm dose of tinidazole or secnidazole. Otherwise, an alternative is metronidazole 200 mg three times a day for 5–10 days.

Reliance on self administered antibiotics carried as part of an "emergency medical kit" gives patients a false sense of security. They are effective only if the diagnosis of bacterial diarrhoea is correct. Inadequate antibiotics can increase the susceptibility to resistant bacteria. They are ineffective against viruses and parasites. Prophylactic antibiotic consumption does not decrease the frequency of diarrhoea. It may instead confound the diagnosis.

Bismuth subsalicylate tablets can be taken prophylactically as 2 tablets 4 times a day for up to 3 weeks for the prevention of traveller's diarrhoea. Though it is fairly effective and is not an antibiotic, it reacts with some other medications. It is not freely available in India.

Most diarrhoeas can be prevented with attention to hygiene and hand washing.

Chapter 5

Jaundice — The Yellow Disease

French physicians in the 19 th century noticed that some people turned yellow when they fell ill. They called this appearance "jaune." The British corrupted this descriptive term to "jaundice", a term still used today.

The course of jaundice varies in different individuals depending on the cause. Many recover completely, others bloat, some waste away and a few die. This difference in the patient response made physicians realize that jaundice is a sign seen in many disease processes and not a diagnosis in itself. They stopped relying on their clinical skills alone. They developed and used laboratory tests and imaging to reach a diagnosis and evaluate the cause of jaundice so that appropriate treatment could be given. A "hit or miss" approach is alright for sports and games, not medical conditions affecting human lives.

Moreover, all people who appear yellow are not jaundiced. Sometimes the appearance of the normal skin colour is altered by fluorescent lighting. There may be an excess of carotene deposited in the skin as a result of consumption of orange-yellow fruits and vegetables like papayas and carrots. Fat deposits under the sclera of the eye or excessive exposure to dust can give dark skinned individuals a "muddy sclera" and a false "jaundiced" look.

The yellow colour in jaundice is actually due to staining of the eyes and skin by the deposition of a pigment called bilirubin. If bilirubin is excreted in excess, there is an obvious colour change in the urine and sweat as well.

Bilirubin is a pigment produced when old red blood cells are broken down in the spleen and liver. It is then metabolized in the liver and excreted. The human eye can discern the yellow colour imparted by bilirubin when the level is three times normal or > 3mg/dl in the blood.

If the number of red blood cells destroyed is greater than normal, the liver is unable to cope with the overload of pigment released and the person becomes jaundiced.. This occurs in some hereditary blood disorders like thalassaemia, and sickle cell disease. Sometimes it due to a hereditary metabolic defect like G6PD deficiency. It may be due to an infection like malaria, or an adverse drug reaction.

Sometimes, the liver cells themselves are defective and unable to cope with the normal amount of bilirubin produced in the body. This occurs in certain hereditary conditions like the Dubin Johnson syndrome. Several members of a family are affected, the jaundice is mild and fluctuating, and it is not fatal.

Immaturity of the liver cells in a newborn, or a mother- baby blood group incompatibility (Rh, ABO) can cause a self limited treatable jaundice in the new born. This progressively worsens with each successive pregnancy. Injections of immunoglobulin (Rho gam) are given to the mother within 72 hours if there is Rh incompatibility to prevent the next baby from being affected. There is no immunoglobulin available for ABO incompatability.

Infection can cause a temporary dysfunction of the liver cell enzymes. The commonest infections are due to the hepatitis viruses A, B, C, D, E. Other infections are caused by the herpes virus, leptospirosis, cytomegalovirus or severe bacterial sepsis can also cause jaundice.

Alcohol is a direct toxin poisonous to the liver cells. Consumption on a regular basis over many years can damage the liver and cause jaundice followed by cirrhosis, hepatic coma and death. Some medications can also cause acute and chronic damage to liver cells. Mouldy raw peanuts contain aflotoxin which is toxic to liver cells and can cause jaundice in people who eat them without roasting or boiling.

Drainage of adequately metabolized normal quantities of bilirubin from the liver may be prevented by blockage of the ducts due to stones, strictures or cancerous deposits. In this case the formation of bilirubin is normal but it cannot drain out.

All jaundice is not the same and cannot be treated alike. Evaluation of jaundice therefore requires a medical and family history, examination, investigation and imaging to reach a correct biochemical and anatomical diagnosis. However, rest and a "liver sparing" diet low in fats and protein helps in most forms of jaundice. The herb phyllanthus ground and swallowed , or administered as an extract is helpful in some self limited non obstructive forms of jaundice.

Jaundice due to viral hepatitis A is the commonest form of jaundice in young adults, and 80 % of the jaundice in them is due to this infection. It recovers spontaneously in a few weeks. Quackery and miracle cures abound, as this infective jaundice is self limited any way. In these cases any "miracle cure" will be successful as the disease process itself is time bound. The tragedy is that people chase after quacks and invest in natural remedies. This means while some other treatable forms of jaundice are not diagnosed, investigated, treated or tackled till it is too late.

Secondary jaundice recovers once the causative factor is removed. Abstaining from alcohol and discontinuing offending drugs may reverse jaundice. If a correctable obstruction is seen on scanning or laparoscopy, surgical treatment provides relief.

Hepatitis A and B are preventable diseases. Vaccination against hepatitis B is offered in a 3 dose schedule before the age of 1 year. Hepatitis A vaccines are a given after the age of 2 years as a 2 dose schedule. This makes the total number of injections for the prevention of jaundice, 5 not 3.

Hepatitis B and C can be severe, relapsing, fatal or chronic. Newer curative treatments with interferon and liver transplants are available and can prolong life. Hepatitis E is a mild self limited jaundice. However it can be fatal in pregnant women.

Before embarking on a course of treatment, it is advisable to obtain a precise documented diagnosis after proper evaluation from a qualified medical person. Jaundice requires appropriate treatment, which depends on a correct diagnosis for that particular type of jaundice. If this is delayed through ignorance or fear, the severity of the illness may increase or even be fatal.

Chapter 6

Syndrome X – The X Factor

"Eat to live—do not live to eat."

Look around as you drive or walk. In India, we have an epidemic of paunches, with a majority of the population, from school children to the elderly affected. The traffic policeman rests his belly on the convenient railing, the truck driver pushes his seat well back, and business people are forced to buy spacious gas guzzling cars to accommodate themselves and their families. As a nation we seem to be marching to our collective destiny leading with our protuberant umbilicus and not with our noses!

What happened?

Something changed us, in the twentieth century, from ramrod straight perambulating healthy individuals, into sedentary pot bellied slouching inactive couch potatoes.

Our ancestors ate vegetarian food and practiced yoga, dancing and the martial arts. Stressful events were mainly to do with sustenance, as they battled floods, infectious diseases, famine and starvation. They were careful and meticulous in their food habits. With no refrigeration, preservatives and storage facilities, the food cooked was always "just enough." This meant that if unexpected visitors arrived the family members went a little hungry. No one ever compromised on hospitality. They learnt to adjust and their bodies adapted.

The scenario has changed now. We have suddenly been thrust into an urbanized life of plenty, comfort and little activity. Adequate food is not a problem. Everyone is busy, so we rely on snacked and packaged food, of dubious nutritive value, dense in calories with a high fat content. This is particularly true in the case of school children who are given cream biscuits, cakes and packaged potato chips for their break in school and when they arrive home at tea time. This is often washed down with a fizzy cola, which can only be described as a sweetened, carbonated, chemical containing bottle of useless calories.

We, are as a nation, now manifesting deadly symptoms of "syndrome X" the "metabolic syndrome" in epidemic proportions.

Metabolic syndrome is suspected

- ➤ If an individual has a parent or sibling with diabetes.
- ➤ If the woman became diabetic during pregnancy.
- ➤ If the woman was diagnosed to have the polycystic ovarian syndrome (PCOS).
- ➤ If blood fasting blood sugar levels are elevated, or the glucose tolerance test (GTT) is impaired.
- ➤ If the individual has a BMI more than 23 (BMI = Ht in wt in kg/ht in m2 in kg).
- ➤ If the waist to hip ratio is greater than 1 in men and 0.8 in women (The narrowest part of your waist divided by the widest part of your hips)
- ➤ If the waist measurement is greater than 40 ins in men and 35 ins in women.
- ➤ If the blood pressure is consistently higher than 135/85.
- ➤ If the fasting blood triglycerides are greater 150 mg/dL
- ➤ If the HDL cholesterol is less than 40mgdL in men and 50 mg/dL in women.
- ➤ If there is a prothrombotic (clotting) state or a proinflammatory state (laboratory tests)

The presence of any three or more of these components places the person at risk for syndrome X, and it is associated with an increased risk of developing young early onset heart disease, diabetes, atherosclerotic plaques in the blood vessels and early death.

The risk occurs from the time the abnormalities occur and is not dependent on the age of the person. Young people in their late teens and twenties can go on to develop diabetes, hypertension and heart disease in their early thirties.

Publicity has been given to the dangers of promiscuity leading to the AIDS epidemic and the dangers of cigarette smoking leading to a plethora of illnesses. The government has national programmes to tackle these problems. Yet, this, is biggest epidemic of them all, affecting around 40 % of our adult population has been largely ignored.

Although the majority of the population already carried the gene for this syndrome, it was incompletely expressed and overt manifestation suppressed by the prevailing environmental and social situations. People were physically active and many were calorie deficient.

Our changing world has made it a rampant preventable disease. Life style modifications are required urgently to prevent a sudden permanent decline in the numbers of our young economically productive adults.

The cause of this metabolic derangement is not known with certainty. All the affected individuals however have insulin resistance, as a result of which the insulin produced in the body does not do its job efficiently.

It is partially triggered by constant unrelieved stress, which in turn is believed to pay an important role in the deposition of abdominal fat. This then triggers the other abnormalities in a cascade.

Tackling the insulin resistance attacks the beginning of syndrome X. The most effective way to do this is increased physical activity and weight loss. An attempt to maintain weight and waist measurements and BMI as close to normal as possible should be made.

Walking as little as 30 minutes every day will reduce insulin resistance. (It also reduces stress levels) For ideal benefits, and to loose weight, initially an hour combined with caloric restriction is probably required.

Weight lifting and other gym exercises do not really help if done alone. They have to be combined with aerobic activity. Also spot reduction of abdominal fat alone, with crunches and other abdominal exercises to correct the ratio alone is not possible without overall weight loss.

Caloric restriction can be achieved by reducing the amount eaten at each meal by 25%. Instead of 3 iddlies, chappatis, dosais eat 2, and do not return for a second helping no matter how mouth watering the food is. Pausing between mouthfuls to a count of twenty and chewing slowly have been shown to reduce intake. Reading, watching television and other mind diverting activities during meal times increases caloric intake.

Try to fill up on fruits and vegetables. These are high in dietary fibre. This will produce a feeling of satiety and eventually reduce total caloric intake

Snacking should be discouraged. Children in particular should have their television viewing curtailed. Cartoons and other programs should not be viewed for more than an hour a week. Televisions should not be viewed at all before the age of two. Reading, watching television and other mind diverting activities during meal times subtly increase caloric intake.

Healthy eating and exercise habits have to be ingrained from childhood, started young and continued forever. Since concerned authorities are not taking this particular devastating epidemic seriously enough, it is up to us as concerned individuals to lead by example. We have to each our children correct food habits and encourage exercise.

Catch them young, feed them correctly, train them right and then turn them loose.

Once a child is shown the path to follow he will not detour from it.

Chapter 7

Diabetes

People often say,

"How can my child have diabetes?"

"How can I get diabetes? I do not eat sweets!"

"No one in my family has diabetes!"

"Everyone in my family has diabetes, what can I do?"

These words are common. A diagnosis of diabetes is frightening, and made more so by many misconceptions about the disease. Fear makes people react with anger, disbelief or denial. This is especially true if the patient is a young child, although it is the commonest endocrine disease affecting children. To the lay person there is something unbelievable about a child developing diabetes.

Sugar is needed by the body for energy. We function best when our blood sugars stay within the normal range. All forms of food (carbohydrates, fats and protein) once digested, is metabolized and eventually converted into "sugar." This enters the blood stream and is taken to all the organs of the body where it is used to provide cells with the energy they require to function. Any excess sugar is taken to the liver and eventually stored as fat for use later if required.

We all have a gland called the pancreas which produces the hormone insulin. This is secreted in controlled quantities to maintain the blood sugar levels in a constant normal range. As the sugar rises more insulin is produced reduce the levels and keep it normal. Unfortunately, insulin production fails in some individuals. This can occur suddenly at any age. Usually it occurs gradually as we grow older. Obesity can render secreted insulin insufficient. In others, the insulin secreted is inefficient or rendered ineffective by antibodies blocking its action. If the insulin available is less than 20 % of the normal then signs of diabetes appear. The commonest are increased appetite and thirst, and weight loss.

In some adults, and overweight inactive diabetic adolescents, the inadequate production of insulin in the body can be boosted with tablets. Once the production is increased, the high sugars become controlled.

In children and in some adults with diabetes, there is no insulin production at all as the pancreas totally fails. They are "insulin dependent" diabetics. Treatment with tablets fail as insulin release cannot be boosted in the absence of production. Such individuals are found to have a higher incidence of some genetic markers, and in many cases the diabetes runs in families. Others may have had their pancreas surgically removed. Diabetes can also develop after infection with measles, mumps German measles or the coxsackie viruses. These infections destroy the insulin producing islet cells in the pancreas.

Insulin is destroyed by the enzymes in the stomach. It cannot therefore be taken as tablets. It has to be administered as injections two or three times a day in the arm, thigh or abdominal wall. Even young patients can be taught to inject themselves as technological advances have made the injections painless. Tiny sharp short disposable needles resembling pens or "guns" can be used for self injection. Recently research is being done to develop a nasal spray of insulin which can be inhaled.

To maintain perfect control, an insulin dependent diabetic should live life with military precision, never varying the quantity of food eaten (no food binges). Diabetics should try never to "go back for a "second helping!" Nor can they vary the activity level. No saying "I am too tired to walk today, I will walk double the distance tomorrow". Practically, it is possible to lead a regimentalized life, but it requires a great deal of mental discipline.

Appetite varies from day to day. Some factors cannot be controlled or factored in. Unforeseen circumstances or travel may prevent regular exercise. We all tend to underestimate calories consumed and overestimate expenditure with activity.

The dose of the insulin required varies and is an equation of the calorific value of the total amount of food eaten, and an estimate of the energy expenditure till the next meal. 8–10 units are required for 500 calories of food. An hour or aerobic activity (running, jogging, swimming) burns up around 300–400 calories, while housework and other stationary activity utilizes 60 calories an hour.

Charts with the calorific value of Indian foods are available with dieticians, in books or can be downloaded off the internet. An estimate of the calorific value of the food on the plate can then be made. An easy way to calculate is to remember equivalents. 1 iddly = 1 chappati= ¾ cup cooked rice= 1 orange/apple. The diet should contain around 1500 calories/day

The blood sugar level can be physically checked before each meal. Computerized "home" glucometers are readily available. They are now relatively inexpensive and the poke is painless. This helps in tighter control of the diabetes and compensates for human error.

In uncontrolled diabetics, the persistently high blood sugar damages internal organs like the kidneys, eyes and heart. Blood supply to the legs can get compromised causing loss of function. Ordinary infections become frequent, uncontrolled and life threatening.

If the food taken has been inadequate or activity excessive, the bloods sugar levels may suddenly drop. This is dangerous. It causes some classic warning symptoms which should be recognized by the diabetic, relatives and friends. It may be a sudden feeling of tiredness, uncontrolled yawning, or an inability to think or speak clearly. There may be sweating and pallor. Later, there may be sweating, twitching, fainting or seizures. This is dangerous and should be tackled immediately by eating or drinking something sweet. Preferably carry a sweet at all times.

Diabetics should exercise 45 minutes a day, reduce their fat intake, and maintain the calorific value that they have been advised. In addition, regular yoga and meditation can help to reduce stress, frustration and depression associated with the disease. This in itself will help to keep the sugars in control.

Diabetes can be controlled but not cured. There is no miracle cure for diabetes. Sugars can be maintained within normal limits with diet and exercise alone, without recourse to medication in some diabetics. Even with a hereditary predisposition to develop diabetes, the onset can be delayed by 10 years or more by maintaining ideal body weight and a healthy active lifestyle.

Management and control of diabetes is not time bound, unlike a fever or infection which recovers in a few days. It means a lifetime of discipline and control. Successful treatment involves lifestyle changes and discipline. Responsibility for sugar control rests with the patient, not with the physician or relatives.

It is important for everyone to understand the disease so that we can all help to provide the resources and support required for our diabetics.

Chapter 8

High Blood Pressure, Angina and Heart Disease

The panic-stricken young engineer stood in front of the doctor's office waiting for his pre employment check up. His heart was pounding and his palms were sweaty. He could actually feel blood rushing to his head. He felt giddy and faint. The room started to swirl around. The symptoms worsened as the white-coated doctor tied on the blood pressure cuff. Not surprisingly, the blood pressure recorded was disproportionately high.

Approximately 10% of the young adult population develops these classical symptoms of "white-coat" hypertension. The sight of the doctor is enough to send the pulse racing and the blood pressure rising. Repetition of the stress causes a recurrence of the symptoms. Fortunately, the hypertension is labile, reversible, and disappears spontaneously once the precipitating stress factor is removed. (In this case the doctor).

Unfortunately most of us are not that lucky.

Hypertension is defined by the WHO is a value of more than 140/90 on three separate occasions. It affects 40% the adult population. Younger men show a slightly higher incidence initially, but the number of affected women increases after the age of fifty, till the ratio becomes equal. This is because of the onset of menopause around that age and the natural decline in the levels of the of the protective female sex hormones.

Tests need to be done if hypertension suddenly appears before the age of 30 or after the age of 55. Secondary causes of hypertension have to be ruled out. It may be due to benign or malignant tumours in the adrenal glands or a "pheochromocytoma" elsewhere. Malfunctioning glands may release steroid hormones and elevate the blood pressure. There may be a congenital narrowing of the aorta (coarctation) or renal artery (stenosis). All these can be surgically tackled. Once the causative factor is removed the blood pressure returns to normal.

Pregnancy can cause a temporary reversible hypertension called pre-eclampsic toxaemia in 7–10 %of women. It is commoner in younger women and during the first pregnancy. It can be severe and fatal to mother and child if improperly managed. The pressure usually reverts to normal after delivery. It usually does not recur in subsequent pregnancies.

Some medications, especially steroids and hormones, prescribed for other illnesses may elevate the blood pressure. The estrogens present in the oral contraceptive pill, or administered as a part of hormone replacement therapy effects idiosyncratic individuals. This iatrogenic (medially caused) hypertension is reversible once the offending agent is withdrawn.

If the cause can be detected and corrected, the hypertension may be reversible.

After the age of forty check your blood pressure every six months to detect primary hypertension. It is a silent asymptomatic killer disease.

The key word is silent. Hypertension can creep up with no signs at all. The commonly touted headache, fatigue, giddiness, palpitations and blurring of vision do not usually appear as early symptoms unless there is a sudden high elevation of the blood pressure. These subjective symptoms cannot be used by the patient to self-medicate and control hypertension. Unfortunately, patients do not understand this and vary their anti-hypertensive medication doses from day to day based on "stress" anger and perceived "tension."

Symptoms of hypertension appear insidiously as a result of vascular changes compromising the blood supply of target "end organs," In the kidney it precipitates renal failure. In the brain it causes paralysis (strokes) and in the heart it causes "heart attacks."

Primary hypertension is inherited and there is a familial predisposition. Obesity, diabetes and high cholesterol and triglycerides predispose to essential or primary hypertension. There are conflicting reports debating whether this is genetic or environmental. Also studies have shown that in families were several members have hypertension have a higher salt intake. Their salt threshold is higher and overall consumption greater. Their taste buds respond to a higher level of salt and the intake automatically tends to be high. Additional salt is often added to food after cooking, and salty snacks are consumed. This should be avoided. Measure out a level teaspoon of salt (5 gms) and then use it to season all the food cooked and consumed by the entire family for the whole day (24 hours). As our food naturally has a high sodium content this is a good way to reduce salt intake. Reduction of salt intake brings down the blood pressure. This is the first step towards control.

Hypertension can be controlled but not cured. It is a disease precipitated and worsened by a stressful lifestyle. Certain life style modifications definitely reduce the blood pressure. It can also decrease the number and dosage of medications taken. This in itself improves the quality of life.

➢ If you have a risk factor like a family history of hypertension, diabetes or high cholesterol correct the biochemical defects.

➢ Weight should be controlled as BMI over 25 increases the severity of the hypertension. Make a serious effort to reduce excess weight and maintain it at a reasonable level. .

➢ Aerobic activities like walking, running, cycling and swimming reduce hypertension. They also improve blood supply to the heart, and hence reduce the incidence of heart attacks. It is never too late and you are never too old to start.

➢ Pressures in the workplace and tension in the family causes stress. Continuous stress leads to hypertension. This is now a normal part of the successful professional urban lifestyle. Usually neither can be changed. Yoga or some other form of meditation practiced daily for 10 to 20 minutes helps people to cope with stressful interpersonal relationships and job insecurities.

➤ If anti-hypertensive medication is advised, it should be taken regularly. Start with one medicine, and after the maximum dose has been reached without side effects add on another if needed.

➤ Timing is important. Tablets should be swallowed at a fixed regular convenient times on schedule with no dangerous memory lapses. They should not be taken in the morning today and evening tomorrow. As far as possible diuretics should be swallowed in the mornings to avoid sleep disruptive night time visits to the toilet.

A high blood pressure eventually has a detrimental effect on the heart. Our heart is the centre of our universe. Without its constant untiring pumping action night and day, the blood supply to the vital control centres in our brain would get cut off, and we would die.

In order for the heart pump to function efficiently, it is supplied with blood and energy through the coronary arteries. These lifelines have to be kept patent and adequate for optimal functioning.

The coronary arteries gradually get blocked as we get older, with fatty deposits or plaques. Some times these break of for get dislodged. They may form clots which get stuck in the smaller blood vessels of the heart compromising the blood supply to that area. This causes characteristic pain called angina.

On television, the angina is dramatic, with the affected individual (usually a man) clutching his chest and falling to the ground. This is a fallacy. Angina is usually not that dramatic ad it is not confined to men.

It may be a heavy, tight, gripping, dull aching discomfort in the centre of the chest, radiating to the jaw, back or arms, which appears during physical activity. It may be associated with fear and sweating. It can be confused with pain due to indigestion, lung disease or pain in the bones of the chest.

If the angina is stable, it is fairly predictable and appears with the same level of activity each time and disappears on rest.

If the pattern of angina changes, and it appears while lying down, or at night , or at rest, the angina has become "unstable," And this is more dangerous.

Angina is investigated with a resting ECG and an exercise ECG. After that, the cardiologist may proceed to echocardiography, to rule out valve defects and other conditions that can precipitate angina.

A coronary angiography is usually the next step. It is a safe, but not totally risk free procedure. It is performed by inserting a thin tube through an artery in the arm or leg and then guiding it into the heart. Dye is then injected into the arteries around the heart. X-rays are then taken which will show it if any of the arteries that supply the heart are blocked.

Angiography helps to establish a diagnosis in angina that is refractory to medical treatment and delineate the exact position of a block. It is used to evaluate abnormal coronary vessels in young patients with angina, especially if there is also a family history with several affected members.

Once a block has been discovered, PTCA (percutaneous transluminal coronary angioplasty) can be done to relieve the block. A balloon mounted on the tip of a long thin catheter is guided under fluoroscopy and used. It can be combined with the insertion of stents to keep the vessels open.

CABG (coronary artery bypass grafting) is used in patients unsuitable for PTCA, and still symptomatic after maximum and optimal medication.

Some of the factors responsible for coronary disease like a genetic predisposition, a positive family history, increasing age and male sex cannot be modified. Others can be changed with a little effort .

- ➤ Purchasing and smoking death facilitating cigarettes and beedis causes 20% of the deaths in men and 17% of the deaths in women due to coronary artery disease. The risk falls by 25% on quitting.
- ➤ A BMI (wt in kg divided by the height in meter squared) over 30 causes 5% of the deaths due to heart disease. Fat

concentrated around the stomach (central obesity) in an unsightly paunch is the most dangerous type of obesity.

➤ A high cholesterol with elevated high density lipoproteins and triglycerides, whether familial or acquired, is associated with a high risk of heart disease.

➤ Uncontrolled untreated high blood pressure reduces the efficiency and perfusion of the heart pump.

➤ Diabetes, either overt or biochemical not only independently increases the risk of heart disease, it compounds the risk posed by other factors.

People sometimes say, "My doctor told me to drink."

Alcohol is protective against heart disease in both men and women. Consumption of around 2 units a day with no "binges" offers some protection. Uncontrolled increased consumption is detrimental.

Certain life style modifications can reduce the incidence of angina and improve the condition of the blood vessels once heart disease has set in.

➤ Maintain body weight as close to the ideal as possible with the BMI between 25 and 30.

➤ Control medical conditions like diabetes and hypertension with regular checkups, dietary modifications and prescribed medications.

➤ Reduce the fat intake and maintain "fat" parameters in the blood as close to normal as possible with medications.

➤ Stop smoking.

➤ Exercise aerobically (walking, jogging, swimming) for at least 30 minutes 4–5 times a week.

You might feel, "It cannot happen to me."

It can and it might, given the present epidemic of diabetes and obesity and our unhealthy stressful inactive lifestyles.

Save yourself! Walk and meditate your way to a lower blood pressure and a better life.

Chapter 9

Piles

Bleeding from anywhere is frightening and blood from the anal area even more so. Drops of blood may appear in the toilet, clothing may be stained, the motion nay be streaked with blood or there may be a sudden profuse external bleed. Patients wince and then say "Help! Do I have piles?"

This fear is increased by gory detailed descriptions of surgical interventions for piles, resulting in rectal incontinence, motion stained clothes, indescribable pain and misery at the hands of unfeeling doctors.

Bleeding from the rectum is a very common complaint and unfortunately patients consider all bleeding from the rectum piles. Some, afraid that doctors will recommend painful, distressing and embarrassing surgery prefer to go to practitioners of alternative medicine. They are not difficult to find. Lurid posters can be found in public places offering non surgical treatment for piles. They posters have a comforting quality about them. It almost seems like a stop-cork is going to be applied to the bleeding area and then all will be well!

Patients who complain of piles actually mean to say, "I passed blood in the toilet". This might have been spontaneous, or an isolated occurrence associated with passage of a hard motion. Passing blood may be painful or painless.

All bleeding from the anal area is not due to piles. Bleeding is a symptom, the cause of which needs to be investigated. It is not a disease in itself. Treating the cause relieves the symptom. If the disease is treated the bleeding will stop.

In alternative systems of medicine there is no diagnosis and an universal remedy is offered for all rectal bleeding. This may not be appropriate if the bleeding is due to another cause like liver disease, a bleeding disorder or cancer. In fact, treating undiagnosed rectal bleeding universally with herbs may be dangerous.

Even though there are many causes of rectal bleeding, the most common cause is piles. The medical name for piles is haemorrhoids. These are actually dilated veins in the rectal area. If they are outside the anus they can be felt soft bumps. They are easily compressible and painless. Sometimes the thin skin over them tears and produces fresh red blood. This can be frightening. Occasionally the haemorrhoids become thrombosed (the blood inside clots). The pile now fells hard and is painful. Internal piles or haemorrhoids are situated higher up and are not visible on the outside. Both types of piles, internal and external are aggravated by chronic constipation and during pregnancy.

Fissures form when the thin skin lining the anus is torn by the passage of a hard stool. The nerve endings and blood vessels are then exposed. Defecation produces excruciating pain and blood, likened to passing barbed wire. This causes the anal sphincter muscles to go into spasm aggravating the condition further.

An abnormal communication tract called a fistula can develop between the rectum and the skin of the anus. It may become infected and painful and discharge discoloured material. This may be an isolated occurrence. It may be due to an infectious disease like TB. It can occur as a complication of chronic diseases like diverticulosis or colitis. It may be part of an autoimmune disease like ulcerative colitis. In all these, the rectum and colon become inflamed, ulcerated and then bleed.

As age advances areas of the rectal mucosa can become weak. These regions can suddenly balloon out and produce a massive bleed.

Profuse diarrhoea with straining can cause part of the rectum to protrude out as a red mass called a prolapse, which bleeds. Sometimes prolapse can occur spontaneously in older individuals as a result of laxity and loss of tone and of the rectal muscles.

Unnatural, abnormal and uncontrolled growth of the rectal mucosa in any age group can produce single or multiple growths called polyps. They may be genetic and inherited. Polyps may occur in many members of predisposed families. These can bleed profusely. They can become cancerous.

All cases of rectal bleeding should therefore be carefully evaluated, especially as cancer of the rectum is a very real possibility. A visual inspection of the rectal area should be followed by a digital rectal examination, then a proctoscopy, sigmoidoscopy or colonoscopy. The site of bleeding can be visualized and biopsied if necessary. X ray procedures like a barium enema should then be done if required.

Most internal and external haemorrhoids and fissure in the early stages respond to simple measures.

- ➢ Take a basin of warm water, and place a crystal of potassium permanganate in it. The water will turn pink. Sit in it for ten minutes twice a day. This will reduce the swelling and relieve pain.
- ➢ Take a stool bulking agent like ipsagol husk regularly till the symptoms subside. This prevents constipation and straining.
- ➢ A local anaesthetic ointment applied before passing motion relives the pain.

Surgery is required for

- ➢ Some large thrombosed or bleeding haemorrhoids.
- ➢ Fistulas, polyps, prolapse and cancer.

Techniques have advanced, and with the use of newer methods, like cauterization, ligation and laser surgery, the morbidity is reduced and treatment is fairly painless.

With alternative treatment, sometimes a mixture of herbs is inserted into the rectum, or the piles are tied off with a string. This cuts off the blood supply causing the piles to shrivel. Problems may develop because the treatment options offered are the same irrespective of the diagnosis. If herbs are inserted in colitis, or if part of a prolapse or cancerous growth is tied, it can lead to complications. Infection may occur because of unsterile techniques. Herbs may be mixed with steroids and administered either as oral pellets or inserted into the rectum. The non- therapeutic unregulated use of steroids may be dangerous.

Spending time and money to reach a diagnosis before embarking on treatment is prudent and wise. With alternative systems of medicine or with no investigations at all, it is not possible to arrive at an anatomic diagnosis. Successful treatment is more likely if there is a correct diagnosis.

The gastro intestinal tract remains healthy with regular habits. This in turn can be achieved with a diet containing sufficient fibre, drinking 3 litres of water a day, and exercising aerobically (walking, jogging or cycling) for 40 minutes a day six days a week.

Yoga and abdominal crunches also maintains the abdominal muscles tone, holding the intestines in place, preventing bloating and ensuring regular bowel habits.

Prevention is prudent and more pleasant than treatment.

CHAPTER 10

SEIZURE DISORDERS

The teenager uttered a hoarse cry and then slid to the floor foaming at the mouth and jerking his arms and legs. An elderly woman stepped forward and tried to force an iron key into his clenched fists. Bystanders offered incomprehensible advice and one threw glass of water on the unfortunate victim.

All these are totally futile actions, as epilepsy, contrary to popular opinion, is not controlled by magnetic fields or prevented by clutching metal. Seizures are caused by a sudden uncontrolled self-limited alteration of the electrical activity in the brain, which is above the 'seizure threshold' for that person. It is not due to sudden possession by evil spirits or eating "cold " food items.

Epilepsy means "seizure." It is the scientific name for a "fit". To label a person "epileptic," there should have been two or more seizures in the preceding six months, without an obvious precipitating cause.

There are many reasons for seizures:

There may be a genetic predisposition.(30 % of the epileptics have a close relative with seizures).

The brain structure itself may have abnormalities producing alterations in the electrical pathway. These may be developmental, or acquired as a result of trauma and surgery. Sudden seizures in a previously normal individual can be a result of :

- ➢ Tumours in the brain.
- ➢ Excessive alcohol consumption or sudden withdrawal.
- ➢ Use of illegal recreational drugs.
- ➢ Low blood sugars and other metabolic or electrolyte imbalances.
- ➢ Disturbances in the blood supply to the brain as a result of "stroke."

➢ Infections of the brain like encephalitis, meningitis and abscesses.

Seizures can be precipitated by physical factors like flickering lights, sleep deprivation or music in a predisposed individual.

"Febrile seizures" during an episode of fever, can occur in 3–4 % of otherwise normal children from the age of 9 months to five years. This does not cause seizure disorders in adult life.

Investigations for epilepsy include blood tests, EEG, CT scan and/or MRI. A person with epilepsy can have a normal brain scan. The EEG may be normal In between attacks. It can however predict whether the seizures are likely to recur or if there is an obvious precipitating factor.

All seizures are not generalized, dramatic and associated with abnormal movements as the one described above. A sudden temporary interruption in the electrical pathways may affect consciousness, awareness, movements or bodily posture. This can result in unfocussed staring (absence attacks), or "feelings" jamais vu (unreality) or déjà vu (familiarity) or disturbances in vision, hearing and balance.

If, despite extensive investigation, no cause for the seizures can be found, they are labelled "idiopathic." There is 50% chance of recurrence of a seizure in 6 months if it is not treated.

With compliance and correct and adequate medication seizures are adequately controlled in 75 % of the patients. Recovery usually occurs in 3 to 5 years if there is no underlying uncorrectable structural brain abnormality or disease.

Once the diagnosis of epilepsy has been made:

➢ Treatment should be regular and taken at the correct time. This means taking medication at the same time every day. Even if you prefer to take medication with food, eat a biscuit or a banana and swallow the medication on schedule if meals are likely to be delayed or missed.

➢ Dosage schedules must be strictly followed.

> ➤ Medications should be tapered and never abruptly discontinued.

In all patients, medications are designed to raise a person's seizure threshold. Brain cells are prevented from sending excessive and confused electrical signals. It increases resistance to having seizures and prevents the seizures from getting started.

The medications used and the treatment has to be individualized. There is no magic drug to treat all seizures in everyone. Some respond well to one medication, others to another. The dosage and drug combinations used also differ depending on the type of seizure, the area of the brain from which it arises, the age and occupation of the person.

People with seizures can lead normal lives. It is illegal to issue a driving license to a person who has had a seizure in the past one year. Photosensitive seizures triggered by flickering or flashing lights may cause difficulties with driving, the use of televisions, computers and fluorescent lights. Some professions like driving heavy vehicles, trains, piloting a plane or steering a ship are unsuitable unless the person has been seizure free for 10 years.. Vocational counselling should be offered to people suffering from seizures. Their academic performance need not suffer if they are managed well

Accidents such as burns, cuts, head injuries can be avoided by making the home and work environment as safe as possible. Elementary safety precautions like avoiding unguarded heights, water and fires should be followed.

Women with epilepsy form a particularly vulnerable segment of the population. Fluctuating levels of the natural hormones during the course of a normal menstrual cycle can cause an increase in the incidence and frequency of epileptic attacks. This may necessitate adjustment of the dose increasing it just before the periods. Fertility is not affected by seizures unless the epilepsy itself is part of some larger endocrine abnormality. However women with seizures are often discriminated against in their own families and after marriage. Although they can lead normal lives and bear children, families arranging an alliance are often unwilling to voluntarily take on this extra liability. The fact that they suffer from seizures is concealed by the marriage broker and the family. During and after the marriage, the woman has to conceal the tablets and swallow them. This means dosage schedules become irregular and the tablets may be discontinued altogether. If a seizure occurs at this time, the woman is often taken by her in-laws to a new doctor. The previous history, investigations and diagnosis are often concealed. A new regimen is embarked upon which may not suit the patient. Recurrence of the seizures may be dangerous.

Transparency about pre-existing medical conditions is safer and better, but may not be practical in our society.

Women with epilepsy who wish to space their families have to be aware that some of the drugs used to treat epilepsy (with the exception of sodium valporate) reduce the efficacy of oral contraceptives. They might become pregnant while on regular treatment with OCPs. A combination pill containing at least 50 mg of oestrogen is effective and can be used. Instead of these higher dose pills, barrier contraception (condoms, diaphragm) or an IUCD (copper T) may be a better option.

During pregnancy, good seizure control should be achieved for the safety of both the baby and the mother. The overall risk of bearing a child with birth defects in an epileptic woman is around 7% as against 3 % in the general population. If a woman planning to become pregnant, she should immediately start folic acid supplements (5 mg /day) when the decision to become pregnant is taken. Folic acid is well documented to have a protective effect on brain and spinal cord development in the first 40 days after conception. Vitamin K orally (20 mg/ per day) should also be given in the week before delivery.

Although small amounts of medication cross over in breast milk, epilepsy is not a contraindication to breast-feeding.

Adequately controlled, properly medicated, epileptics can lead normal and productive lives.

CHAPTER 11

MENTAL ILLNESS

An elderly couple stood watching the chaotic traffic. He turned to his wife and said, "The entire world seems mad except me and you." He paused, considered and continued, "and sometimes you seem a little mad too."

His observation was probably not far from the truth. Serious psychotic disorders like schizophrenia, dementia, delusions and paranoia are present in 0.5 % of the population. Mild psychiatric disturbances are present in 20% of the population. In addition, emotions can aggravate or alleviate "real illnesses," leaving no sharp dividing line between the physical and the mental. They tend to overlap and influence each other. This leads to psychosomatic illness where the psyche (mind) influences the soma (body). Almost 60 % of the patients visiting the doctor have stress related or psychiatric illness.

All psychiatric patients are not obviously ill. They do not talk to trees or run naked down the street. There are variations and gradations of the symptoms and manifestations of psychiatric illness as in any other disease process.

Certain families have more members in need of psychiatric care. This has led to postulates that the likelihood of developing such an illness may be inherited, with abnormal personality traits being passed on from the parents. Medical studies in twins and in adopted children, helps to reinforce this claim. Twins separated at birth and reared separately in foster homes with different nurturing environments often develop varying degrees of the same psychiatric illness.

Brain cells communicate with each other by transmitting signals with chemicals called neurotransmitters. A correct balance has to be maintained for a person to function efficiently in society. Injuries to the brain can cause defects in the production, degradation, or the ratio between the various chemicals. This causes manifestations of mental disease.

Damage can occur before birth in the womb, during the birth process itself, or after birth as a result of aging, chemicals or an accident. Mental illness may be triggered in a previously normal person by overwhelming psychological stresses like separation, early untimely death of a parent, extreme neglect, or physical, sexual or emotional abuse. Interplay between various environmental and social factors may then prolong the illness.

Newer scanning techniques have demonstrated that blood flow to certain areas of the brain and even its actual physical size differs in persons with psychiatric illnesses. The chemical reaction (neurotransmitter release) in the brain as a response to day-to-day events is also altered. This is similar to change in the blood flow to the heart muscle and the chemicals released causing damage to the cardiac muscle in heart attacks.. Yet, diabetes, hypertension, heart disease, renal failure or cancers are considered "real" organic diseases. There is no discrimination against people suffering from these ailments. Their families are not ashamed.

Society does not accept mental illness, as a disease of the brain. For centuries psychiatric patients have been referred to derisively as "lunatics". They are the objects of scorn. They are ill-treated, denied their basic human rights, chained, beaten, confined or hidden by their families from society. They are denied treatment. Some are married to unsuspecting partners in the hope that in some mysterious way marriage will cure the illness. Most of these patients would probably readjust to society, with appropriate and timely medical intervention.

General physicians can treat the milder forms like depression, anxiety, panic attacks, somatization, (transfer of symptoms to a part of the body), eating disorders and substance abuse. These may present at only certain times in a persons life. Psychotic illnesses like dementia, schizophrenia, paranoia require expert qualified evaluation and help.

Screening for mild psychiatric illness requires affirmative answers to the questions:

- ➤ "During the past month have you felt down, depressed, hopeless, useless, and experienced no interest or pleasure in any activity?"
- ➤ Or "have you had a recent onset of excessive irrational fatigue, irritability, headaches, chest pains impotence, lack of sex drive or vague stomach symptoms?"
- ➤ A spouse, close friend, relative or caretaker should also have noticed these symptoms.

Depression may occur spontaneously or be precipitated by concurrent illness, death, or some other traumatizing event. The feeling described is one of lethargy, inability to perform day-to-day activities, lack of interest in appearance and a feeling of hopelessness. If it coexists with anxiety, the person appears agitated, and there may be lack of eye contact.

Somatization involves a plethora of medically unexplained symptoms like exhaustion, dizzy spells, intolerance to noise, tingling and unexplained pain in a physically normal adult. The symptoms are not substantiated by physical examination . The investigations all give normal results. Rational treatment offers no relief.

Panic attacks are recognized by the effected individual. They are precipitated and prolonged by hyperventilation and accompanied by sweating and palpitations.

Substance abuse involves alcohol, recreational drugs, smoking or over indulgence in food.

Exercise started at the primary school stage and prolonged into the geriatric age group significantly decreases the incidence and duration of minor psychiatric illnesses. Teenagers interested in fitness and sports do not experiment with banned intoxicating substances. The risk of developing major psychiatric illnesses is also reduced with regular activity. Stress is reduced with a regular structured life.

The ability to cope is better and the incidence of minor psychiatric illnesses is less.

Regular aerobic activities like walking, swimming, cycling or jogging for 45 minutes a day, five to six days a week, have been shown to release endorphins from the muscles utilized. These naturally occurring chemicals elevate the mood, increase energy levels and maintain mental equilibrium. The stresses encountered in the roller coaster of life become easier to handle.

Exercise is free and its benefits are immeasurable.

Start today.

CHAPTER 12

ALCOHOLISM

Tipplers Ahoy !

"A jug of wine, a loaf of bread, — and thou beside me in the wilderness,

Oh wilderness were paradise anew." Omar Khayyam

The drunk asleep on the pavement, oblivious to torrential rain or blazing sun, and the suave educated successful executive, with bulging red eyes, loud laughter and witty conversation both have the same drinking problem, only their social status is different.

Drinking occurs all over the world, and alcohol has been in existence for centuries. . Adults of both sexes and all classes consume liquor either openly or secretly.

Alcohol was initially brewed as toddy from fermenting fruits, vegetables or grains. It was then distilled into the stronger liquor (arrack). All kinds of objects were added to increase the potency of the brew, like waste rubber, old jute and the odd dead insect or two.

Occasionally, unscrupulous vendors added toxic methyl alcohol. This is cheap, colourless and provides a "kick." Unfortunately, it results in blindness and sometimes even death. Politicians usually capitalize on the public out cry that follows, with temporary stop gap measures and financial compensation. The deeper social and psychological problems giving rise to the alcohol addiction and dependence are not tackled. The nexus between the powerful, the police and the arrack vendor remains intact.

Whiskey, rum, brandy, gin vodka, wines and beer are sold in India as a variety of "spirits" known locally as Indian Made Foreign Liquor (IMFL). Grains and fruits are scientifically fermented, cured, aged, purified, distilled, flavoured and bottled hygienically in factories. It is more expensive, as it is also heavily taxed, and out of reach for the common man.

The labourer drinks arrack or toddy, falls on the road or reaches home belligerently to abuse and beat his wife. The businessman's whiskey soon makes his humorous conversation incomprehensible, and he is reduced to a red eyed, drooling, aggravating buffoon, who may then return home to do the same.

People drink socially to relax, forget their worries and cope. This sounds innocuous enough, but 20 % develop alcohol dependence and further 20% become problem drinkers.

Alcohol consumption is out of control, when there is a strong uncontrollable urge to drink, earlier and earlier in the day, accompanied by an inability to stop. The conditioned numbed brain does not emit the satiety or warning signals saying "enough." Stronger and larger drinks are required to achieve the same "kick." For an addict to failure to consume alcohol results in sleeplessness, anxiety, nervousness, hallucinations, tremors and eventually convulsions.

All the organs in the body are affected by addiction to alcohol. It initially produces sweating and flushing. The muscles become weak. Working becomes difficult. The blood pressure becomes unstable; the heart is affected, with dysfunction of the muscles and the electrical conducting system. The liver enzymes are unable to cope, the organ becomes damaged and cirrhosis sets in. This gives rise to jaundice, bleeding from the oesophagus or rectum and fluid collection in the abdomen. Eventually the liver fails to perform its function of detoxification. Poisonous chemicals build up. There may be overwhelming infection resulting in coma and death.

The pancreas can be dangerously inflamed. This gives rise to pancreatitis. The stomach develops ulcers. The absorption, storage and utilization of vitamins become inadequate. There may be tingling and loss of sensation in the hands and feet. Alcohol rapidly suppresses the higher functions of the brain with loss of memory and lack of clear thinking. Eventually there may be hallucinations, convulsions coma and death. Alcohol is called "the great deceiver."

Sexual desire is increased, but the performance is frustratingly below par, often plagued by premature ejaculation or impotence.

Genetics do play a part in determining a susceptibility to alcoholism. Several members of a family for many generations may become alcoholics. The same area of the brain, and genes determine susceptibility both to alcohol and to other substance abuse. However, although it can be inherited, progression to dependence is influenced by availability and environment.

Some alcoholics have an abnormal psychopathic personality that prevents them from logically analyzing action and consequence. Others are depressive and this makes them stubbornly embark on a road to self destruction. Anything becomes an excuse to drink, marital discord, frustration, stress, unhappiness or social pressures.

Urgent help is needed if:

➤ You are unable to cope with your responsibilities at home or work.

➤ People have asked you to stop drinking.

➤ You drink before driving or operating heavy machinery.

➤ Interpersonal relationships at home or the workplace cease to be congenial.

➤ Aggressive behaviour at home or outside has resulted in violence and assault.

➤ If you wake up needing another drink first thing in the morning to quiet the tremors and steady your nerves.

➤ One or more of your organs are biochemically or symptomatically affected.

Alcoholism is a progressive problem that can be fatal. It does not disappear spontaneously with a change in the environment or different friends. New cronies are soon found as "birds of a feather flock together." An arranged marriage with an unsuspecting woman will only add to the problem not cure it.

To stop requires awareness, motivation, determination and action. Family support is invaluable, but it is difficult. Many alcoholics are irritable and irrational. They lack insight into their condition and do not appreciate advice or concern. If the blood relatives find the person intolerable, then how can an unrelated spouse cope?

Help and support is available in specialized detoxification centres, with psychiatrists and with Alcoholics Anonymous (AA) in the major cities.

Alcohol must be stopped abruptly. It cannot be reduced one drink at a time. Gradual reduction results in relapse and failure.

Withdrawal also causes problems. There may be tremors, hallucinations and an unbearable craving. Life may become more stressful, with associated irritation and insomnia.

In addition the battered body, damaged at the cellular level needs to be nourished back to health.

General weakness requires a balanced diet supplemented with vitamins and minerals. If the nerves or heart have been affected high doses may be required, particularly of thiamine and this may have to given by injection.

Acidity can be tackled by eating bland meals at regular intervals. Cigarettes, tea, coffee and hot and spicy food should be avoided. If there is chronic indigestion, bloating and discomfort, tablets may be required.

Jaundice, abdominal distension, pain or bleeding from any site must be taken seriously. Medical help should be immediately sought.

Co-existing diabetes, hypertension and heart disease must be tackled appropriately.

Psychiatric help should be sought for restlessness, agitation, sleeplessness, depression and suicidal thoughts. Anti depressants may be prescribed. Other medications are available to tackle alcoholism and its side effects. They are used to produce an aversion to alcohol. They must be taken continuously, not stopped because a drink is needed. They can produce severe serious side effects if consumed along with alcohol..

Yoga, relaxation therapy, meditation and acupuncture complement conventional medical treatment. Acupuncture can be used to cause aversion. Physical exercise and a regular lifestyle help to provide mental resilience and resist temptation.

The rocky road to abstinence is full of pitfalls. It needs to be traversed steadfastly one step at a time with insight, determination, motivation, medication and loyal support from family and friends.

If there is a family history of alcoholism or substance abuse, do not reach for that first drink.

CHAPTER 13

SMOKING AND NICOTINE ADDICTION

Puffs, Chews, and Snuff

The college girl balanced a filter tipped cigarette between her slender fingers and blew smoke rings nonchalantly at passers by. The teenage boy was dressed in blue jeans and leaning against the railing. He utilized a "hands free" technique with a beedi drooping from the corner of his mouth. She looked sophisticated and he looked like a thin desi version of the Malboro man.

Why do teens get addicted to tobacco at this young age?

Is it due to peer pressure?

Or an appeal to the ego with macho advertising?

Sheer boredom?

A desire to "concentrate" study or fight sleep?

Or a feeling that this was the way to loose weight and appear glamorous?

Recently the government tried unsuccessfully to ban smoking in movies and advertisements on bill boards and hoardings. Movies magazines and bill boards still subtly advocate smoking. We have hoardings of scenes from our vernacular movies, depicting heroes and villains with beedis clenched between their teeth, discarded just before springing into action. Newspapers carry photographs of business tycoons with filter tipped cigarettes or pipes. Tobacco companies (cigarettes, beedis, chewing tobacco and snuff) have developed an effective strategy promoting tobacco use as a glamorous symbol of freedom and independence. Subtly, it is even promoted as an appetite suppressant producing thinness in women (the black coffee cigarette diet for an hourglass shape)!

In short become a thin sophisticated person with bad breath, smelly clothes, yellow teeth and nails, brittle skin, wasted money, and bad health.

Smoking causes heart disease, stroke, multiple cancers, respiratory diseases, and other expensive and chronic illnesses. Women who smoke are more likely to have smaller, sicker babies, be infertile and have more miscarriages. They also have more complications in pregnancy are at greater risk for breast cancer, early menopause and osteoporosis.

Women do not really have to reach out for that first puff. Many are victims of second hand smoke (passive smoking). If the unfortunate victim (usually women and sometimes children) lives in close proximity to a smoker, they also suffer from the same deleterious effects. They have all the side effects without the habit. (All pain and no pleasure).

Tobacco in all forms is addictive. Social norms, or fear of parental retribution force people to pursue the addiction in secret and smoke in bathrooms and balconies. Some resort to the use of tobacco laced snuff, flavoured chewing tobacco or to brushing their teeth secretly with tobacco powder to receive the "nicotine" kick.

Tobacco companies have known about the destructive health effects of tobacco and the addictive power of nicotine for at least 40 years. Light cigarettes and beedis have the same carcinogenic ingredients as regular cigarettes. They all contain lead, ammonia, benzene, DDT, butane gas, carbon monoxide, arsenic, and polonium 210. In addition the menthol and other cooling agents in light cigarettes increase the addiction and carcinogenic effect.

Cigarettes cause more deaths than AIDS, illegal drugs, car crashes, homicides, and suicides combined. As many as one-half of long-term smokers will die of causes related to tobacco, even though it is an easily preventable cause of death and life with disability.

Most young smokers start smoking convinced that they have the willpower to quit whenever they want to, but in actual fact 90 % are still smoking five years later. Many sincerely believe that complications will side step them and effect others!

It is never too late. Smokers who do manage to quit will, on average, live longer and be healthier than those who do not.

All over the world, governments are trying. Advertisements for cigarettes are banned on television, the radio and hoardings. Recently, an attempt has been made to ban smoking in movies. Smoking in public places like trains, buses, offices and educational institutions is against the law. Chewing tobacco has been banned in a few states in India.

Cigarette packets have a statutory warning printed on them. "Cigarette smoking is injurious to health." In a countries where many cannot read English, and will this work?

Conversely, advertising beedis is not against the law in India, and the packets do not carry a statuary warning even though the tobacco contained in them is just as harmful. This is because the beedi caucus is rich and powerful.

In India, the beedi industry is spread over 13 States and 3 Union territories. It employs more than three million workers, males, females and children. . It is dominated by Scheduled Castes, Scheduled Tribes, Backward Tribes and unorganized groups It is one of the industries employing child labour. The children sit huddled for 14–17 hours a day, rolling beedis with their nimble fingers. They do not go to school. Entire families work rolling filling and packing the beedis. The families, illiterate and often bonded, live in abject poverty and debt. They constitute an enormous vote bank that politicians cannot ignore.

The beedi industry provides income for the workers families, to transporters, and huge profits to the factory owner. This means that while the government has to promote the nations health, highlighting the pitfalls of tobacco utilization, it is constrained by the loss of jobs any stringent action would entail, an inability to provide alternative employment, the loss of revenue as taxes, and alienation of an important vote bank. Hence the government takes a fairly hypocritical stand on tobacco and it is left to the health professionals to sing dirges and tales of woe.

Face-to-face and interactive counselling on a one is to one basis Is very successful in motivating people to quit. Yet, how many health care professionals have the time or Inclination? Counselling an unwilling individual, and listening to arguments is stressful and not financially lucrative.

Medication, the sustained release form bupropion SR, is marketed in India. It is a non-nicotine medication that is thought to reduce the urge to smoke by affecting the same chemical messengers in the brain that are activated by nicotine. It is expensive, the dosage has to be individualized, and it has to be taken for a prolonged period. Motivation and persistence are usually lacking in smokers and it has not been a success in India. Nicotine patches and gum are not available in India.

Anyone who wants to quit has to grit their teeth and "just do it."

The college girl puffed again, "it's not how I visualize myself dying, I can stop if I want to, it is not that hard, I can't get lung cancer. I am a woman and only 20."

Brave words. False assumptions.

CHAPTER 14

ASTHMA AND REACTIVE AIRWAYS

"I'll huff and I'll puff"—

After saying that , if only a whistling sound issues when you try to breathe, or else you have paroxysms of uncontrolled coughing, then you may be part of the 5% of the Indian population with asthma.

Most medical professionals are wary of using the word. They pussyfoot around the diagnosis and call it "allergy" or "eosinophilia" or sometimes even the correct terminology of "reactive airways disease."

Then why is the diagnosis viewed with so much dread?

It is mainly due to a combination of folk lore, myths and circulated horror stories, compounded by the sneaking suspicion that 'asthma' may actually be a synonym for 'tuberculosis'! The two are very different entities, with cough as their only common symptom.

Also, asthmatics in the old movies always died puffing for breath and turning blue. The general public began to equate asthma with debility, enforced inactivity and an early death.

As a disease, asthma can occur at any age. It tends to start in childhood and is more common among boys. The incidence is increasing internationally probably a cumulative effect of increasing population, overcrowding, urbanization and environmental pollution.

It clusters in families, with allergies. Some become 'wheezers', others 'sneezers' and some 'scratchers', depending on where the allergic tendencies has chosen to manifest itself.

The sneezers develop stuffy blocked noses at the slightest provocation. They are unable to breathe and sneeze repeatedly. Sometimes the nasal mucosa itself hypertrophies and forms polyp like masses.

Scratchers itch and scratch till their skin becomes discoloured and hypertrophied. Sometimes they use inappropriate instruments to itch. It becomes a habit, and "the more they itch the more they scratch."

Of the three, the wheezers are the most dramatic, gasping and breathing in short inefficient spurts during an attack. It may be frightening to an emotionally involved family member, and invite unsolicited advice from by standers and well wishers. The recurrence of attacks may be depressing and lead to a search for alternative therapy or quack cures.

All the three are allergic manifestations precipitated by contact with allergens in the environment. These individuals have high levels of a particular immunoglobulin E and also tend to release chemicals like histamine when confronted with any noxious stimulus. The chemicals cause airways to constrict and collapse on one another. As the person attempts to force out the air during breathing a whistling sound ensues. Mucous collects in these blocked tubes forcing them to narrow further. An inability to breathe causes a panic attack which worsens the situation. Initial attacks are reversible and rarely fatal. They can spontaneously resolve. Sometimes exposure to steam can abort an attack.

Asthma is actually caused by allergens with individualized triggers in different people. There are a few common allergens like cockroach dander, mice droppings house mites and dust. Persistent attacks in school or in the work place affecting more than one person warrants a diligent search for allergens peculiar to that environment.

The mosquito breeding season has started with the onset of the monsoon. Vaporizing mosquito repellents (coils, mats, liquids) are popular. Some appear to be odourless and silently fill the environment. They all precipitate wheezing and sneezing in susceptible individuals. Cigarette smoke acts in much the same way.

In short, a clean, chemical free, pest-free house with non-smoking family members will go along way towards preventing wheezing.

If you are allergic and wheeze or sneeze:

> ➤ Please do not stand in line and pay good money to swallow live fish, as advertised in many newspapers and magazines and vouched for by lists of eminent personalities to control wheezing. The benefits are not proven and are questionable.

> ➤ Also, avoid the 'really good' unqualified practitioner who treats with a monthly injection as it is actually a potent long acting steroid preparation. It will definitely offer immediate relief, but once the life of the steroid is over (usually around 21 days), the symptoms recur with renewed virulence causing dependence, and many side effects, like baldness, hirsuitism (in effect it means you'll lose hair on your head but grow it every where else), obesity, hypertension diabetes and osteoporosis.

> ➤ Do not take green herbs ground to a paste. They contain the precursors of drugs previously popular in the treatment of asthma (like ephedrine) in an unpurified form and administered in unregulated dosages. An unscrupulous supplier may mix the herbs with oral steroid preparations to ensure rapid relief.

All these unregulated treatments do offer a "cure" but at a high price to your health. All these treatments offer dramatic cures, but that is simply because asthma itself is episodic, with naturally occurring long (months on end) symptom free intervals.

With a little care, and proper medication asthma is controllable and frequent attacks preventable. One of the methods is orally administered medication. But for the medicine to be effective, it has to reach the lungs from the stomach through the blood. En route, it may produce side-effects, although most drugs used in the treatment of asthma are safe and non-toxic.

A direct delivery system works best with the medicine going straight to the lungs. Many devices are available for this, like spacers, rotahalors, inhalers and nebulizers. These can be loaded with bronchodilators to open out the constricted airways and anti-inflammatory agents to prevent them from closing up again. Once patients are confident about using the devices, and have grasped the principles of treatment, they can control their own bronchospasm best.

Treatment of asthma or reactive airways (as it is medically called), has to individualized. Best results are obtained if the patient is a partner to the treatment. They are the best judge of the adequacy of medication, as early warning signs like a tightening of the chest are subjective and can be picked up only by the patient.

The frequency and severity of attacks can be reduced by regular exercise like fast walking, running, skipping or cycling continuously for a minimum of 20 minutes a day combined with the breathing asanas taught in yoga. And most important, no asthmatic should ever smoke.

Encouraged to use proper medication, taking prophylactic inhaled medicine when required and freed from unsolicited advice, asthma is not frightening and most asthmatics can efficiently manage their disease and lead normal and productive lives.

CHAPTER 15

SNIFFLES AND SNEEZES

The weather improves after the rains, but this welcome change in the climate brings with it an epidemic of "colds." Runny noses, incessant sneezing, fever, body pains and an accompanying headache reduce efficiency and increase absenteeism in school and in the work place.

Over a 100 types of rhinoviruses (rhino is Latin for nose) can cause colds. People gradually develop immunity to the particular attacking rhinoviruses as they recover from a "cold." We come into contact with several species of viruses and most people develop two to three colds a year. Recovery from a cold takes 7 –10 days, if no complications develop. This makes some people feel that they have been "having a cold which lasted the whole year."

Rhinoviruses are spread through the air suspended in droplets during coughing and sneezing. They are directly deposited in the nose from the air or by the contaminated fingers. They can also be deposited in the eye and then travel down the tear duct to the nose. These hardy viruses can also temporarily survive on furniture, walls and clothing until an appropriate susceptible host is found. Hands placed on contaminated walls or furniture and then on the nose enable the virus to gain a foot hold on the respiratory tract.

In these days of centralized air conditioning and closed spaces the incidence of colds is increasing. The virus recirculates in closed spaces looking for susceptible individuals.

Cold viruses deposited in the nose are transported by cilia action to the back of the throat in 10–15 minutes. The nasal mucous membrane attempts to wash out the viruses by swelling up and increasing its secretions. This causes sneezing and drippy noses as the body attempts to rid itself of the infection.

Mothers pass on immunity to rhinoviruses to their children, both in utero and through the breast milk. This partially protects breast fed babies for the first 6 months of life. After that the number of colds increases proportionately depending on the number of people the child is in contact with. Later, as children come into contact with many others, especially in a closed environment like a poorly ventilated classroom, the number of infections proportionately increases. This causes a dramatic increase in the number of fevers, colds and "lost school days" at the primary school level.. Around 8 colds can occur during the first school year in a normal child. As each cold lasts for around a week, this means around 60 days of ill-health due to colds alone.

A rhinovirus infection must be distinguished from "allergic rhinitis." which is not infectious or transmittable. It is a watery response from the nasal mucosa in response to contact with an allergen. It may be seasonal, in which case the person has symptom free intervals in between attacks. It is usually due to particular plant pollen or the cracker bursting Diwali season. Allergic rhinitis may be perennial, when the person has a drippy nose and is sneezing all the year round. This is often precipitated by mosquito mats or repellents, room fresheners and other sprays, agarbathis, incense, sambrani or in school by chalk dust.

Allergies are difficult to treat if the cause is not determined. They can cause swelling of the nasal mucosa and permanent nose block. The newer anti allergic nasal sprays if used regularly as directed for 2–3 months cause the hypertrophied mucosa to shrink and the allergy to subside.

Once the cold process has started, it cannot be aborted and has to run its course. Although no real "cold cure" has yet been discovered, amelioration of the symptoms can be achieved. Treatment regimens that are successful some people do not work for others. It is difficult to evaluate superiority of one regimen over another, as the disease itself is self-limiting.

Nose drops can relieve nasal stuffiness. Commercially available saline nose drops are effective of used every two hours. The head should be tilted well back with the face turned to one side while applying the drops. Advertised "decongestant" or "steroid" nose drops are initially more efficient. However they cause habituation and require an increase in the frequency of application to obtain the same benefit. It becomes difficult to stop using them as the nasal mucosa develops rebound congestion if they are stopped. Eventually the nasal mucosa itself may become atrophic and the sense of smell reduced.

Children should be taught to blow out nasal secretions and not sniff it inside. Handkerchiefs or tissues should be used. Antihistamines reduce sneezing and the irritating nasal drip. They cause sedation and should not be used while driving. They should not be taken with alcohol. Some antihistamines like promethazine are contraindicated in children under the age of 2 years because of sedation and respiratory depression.

Concomitant aches and pains can be relieved with the judicious use of paracetamol, brufen, aspirin or naprosyn.

Saline or aspirin gargles, and steam inhalations relieve sore throats.

If recovery from a cold has not occurred in 7–10 days, or the watery secretions turn purulent and yellow, it usually means that secondary infection or sinusitis has occurred. This responds to appropriate adequate antibiotic therapy. Antibiotics however are not effective against the rhinovirus. Prophylactic antibiotic administration is neither effective nor efficient as it does not reduce the duration of the cold.

The nasal passages of children are shorter straighter smaller and more easily blocked. This predisposes them to complications like bronchitis or ear infection. However their small immature sinuses are usually spared. Ear infection is usually signalled by incessant crying and obvious tenderness if the ear is touched or pulled.

Person to person spread of colds can be prevented if the secretions are not sniffed in, but sneezed out into disposable tissues, which are appropriately discarded. Hands are washed frequently. Eyes are not touched or rubbed even if they itch.

Colds in India spread within communities like wild fire because as a nation we lack civic sense. We send sick children to school. We do not really care abut other healthy uninfected children in the class. Schools too harangue the parents if there are too many school days missed as a result of ill health. Parents sometimes feel that the child gets more rest in the class room than at home as there is prolonged enforced inactivity in school. This means that the cold keeps spreading and the class often sounds like an orchestra sniffing at various pitches! We forget that the teacher and ayah cannot really cope with an irritable unwell child. We do not provide facemasks to prevent droplet infection or encourage the use of tissues.

The ability to cope with a cold is better in people who generally keep themselves fit with regular physical aerobic exercise and the yoga breathing asanas. The number of infections is less. Noses do not get blocked as they are trained to remain open.

Fresh air, a balanced diet and regular exercises reduces the number of colds and generally increases immunity and reduces allergic reactions.

Chapter 16

Pimples—Oh no! Not another one!

Acne affects 75 percent of the adolescent population all over the world. Pimples are one of the causes of adolescent depression, social isolation, and suicide.

It therefore comes as no surprise that treating acne is financially lucrative for physicians, the pharmaceutical industry, homeopaths, cosmetologists, and owners of beauty parlours. Teenagers are willing to go to any lengths and costs to acquire unblemished complexion.

The cause of acne must be understood for any treatment to succeed.

Skin is protected by a naturally occurring oily substance called sebum, which starts to appear at adolescence due to the action of hormones. In some people sebum-filled skin pores mysteriously collapse, become secondarily infected with the bacterium P acnes to form pimples.

The exact cause of acne is not known. Heredity plays a role in the development of acne and hormonal changes precipitate the problem in predisposed individuals. Hormonal imbalances occurring during puberty (children do not have acne), pregnancy, and menopause may worsen acne or cause its sudden appearance. A higher level of male hormones predisposes to acne.

Contact with dandruff, split hair, oil-based make-up and perfumed face powder increases pimples on the face and neck.

Pimples should not be picked, scrubbed or shaved off as this worsens the problem. Contrary to popular belief, lack of bathing or poor hygiene does not increase pimples. Instead, vigorous scrubbing causes breaks in the skin which predisposes to inflammation, pimples, and scarring.

Stress, anxiety, depression, chocolates and oily snacks do not worsen acne directly. All these however predispose to weight gain, which alters and imbalances hormones, leading to acne.

Skin takes at least two months to respond to treatment for acne. Also, as the exact cause of acne is not known, treatment is based on unproven anecdotal "hit or miss" regimens.

In mild cases of acne, creams containing benzyl peroxide (such as Clearasil and Persol) are quite successful. The cream needs to be generously applied twice a day on a clean face for 15 minutes and then rinsed off with water. A small quantity of a gentle moisturiser like baby oil must then be applied. Initial applications may cause redness of the skin if it is exposed to sunlight. It also tends to discolour and bleach dark coloured fabrics.

If this does not work then certain antibiotics may be prescribed in small doses for prolonged periods with a view of eradicating the P acnes bacteria. Antibiotics, though, can produce side-effects., They have to be taken for a long time and the bacteria themselves may become resistant.

Supplements of vitamins and minerals including zinc in therapeutic doses may help.

In women, the hormonal imbalances precipitating acne can be corrected by supplying the hormones artificially in the correct ratio as oral contraceptive pills.

In resistant cases of acne, isotretinoin and its derivatives may be prescribed either as a tablet or an ointment. These have serious side-effects and can cause myalgia (muscle pain) and hair loss as well as precipitate depression. Also, pregnant women can produce abnormal babies or have abortions, so none of the above methods should be used if there is the slightest chance of pregnancy.

Pimples and scars can be removed by relatively expensive procedures like dermabrasion, laser resurfacing, or subincision. Pits and depressed scars can be filled with collagen. Superficially scarred skin can be removed in layers by chemical peels. Several sittings are required for these procedures. It is advisable that these be done only by qualified and experienced dermatologists or plastic surgeons.

At the other end of the cost spectrum, there is the homemade face pack, which can be made of simple inexpensive readily available ingredients. Lemon juice can be mixed with grated cucumber and curd or papaya mixed with honey and curd. This is then washed off after half an hour with a paste made from 500 gms of green gram, 500 gms of masoor dhal and 100 gms of kasturi manjal powdered together. You can then steam your face and moisturise your skin with a mixture of 500 ml sesame oil, 500 ml coconut oil and 100 ml olive oil.

A diet rich in fresh fruits and green leafy vegetables is helpful as it increases the antioxidant and carotenoid content of the food, which in turn keeps the body healthy. They also reduce the caloric content of the food, helping in weight control.

Try to maintain a BMI (weight / height in metre squared) of 25 and walk, jog or run in open air for 30 minutes everyday. Fresh air and regular physical activity relieve stress and correct hormonal imbalances.

The fitness regimen will also give you an inner radiance that shines out and dazzles the world irrespective of facial blemishes.

CHAPTER 17

BODY ODOUR

"Phew! What is that smell?"

Body odour can be offensive to others. It might be the smell of stale sweat in a crowded unventilated area; it may be due to a disease process or just bad breath (halitosis). Often, unfortunately, it is obvious to everyone but the victim who is blissfully oblivious. We are immune to our own smell since our nose has become habituated to it. It is embarrassing, and eventually it drives away friends, family, and sometimes even spouses.

Television advertisement for body talc, deodorant sprays and toothpaste truthfully perpetuate the concept that body odour in any form signals an end to romance, friendship, popularity and togetherness. For once, the advertisements may not be far from the truth.

Each adult has a distinctive recognizable body odour, which is unique. It comes arises from the sweat and sebaceous glands. There are two kinds of sweat glands, the Eccrine and the Apocrine. Sweat from the Eccrine glands found all over the body mainly regulate the body temperature. The Apocrine sweat glands are found in the groin and underarm areas. Sweat is actually initially colourless and odourless. In an airless environment covered with non absorbent clothing, bacteria grow in the sweat. They produce a smell. Odour also comes from the action of bacteria on sebum, a waxy mixture of cholesterol, fatty acids and proteins secreted by the sebaceous glands in the skin. Skin is constantly being replenished, and dead skin itself also forms nutritive food for the bacteria.

Survival in the animal kingdom required a well developed and discriminating sense of smell. Cavemen could identify strangers, prey, predators, and smell fear. As man evolved, the olfactory system (smelling apparatus) became redundant and rudimentary, and now we can recognize only a few basic pleasant and repugnant odours. Smell is a primitive animal instinct, and is still well developed in babies. They can use it to recognize familiar people and to "home in" on the mother's presence. Dogs and some other animals can recognize an individual's smell. This canine talent is used track people, detect illicit drugs and sniff out bombs.

In certain medical illnesses, the body odour changes, becomes distinctive and can be recognized with experience. In liver disease, particularly cirrhosis, and in renal failure there is a musty uricose odour near the patient. Schizophrenics have a distinct odour in their sweat due to a chemical called trans-3-methylhexanoic acid. Some lung diseases (particularly abscesses) smell like apple blossoms. Non healing ulcers due to pressure sores, diabetes or cancer smell like rotting compost. Anaerobic bacteria producing an infection anywhere in the body emit a pungent repugnant odour. Advanced cancer has a distinctive smell. Urinary tract infection makes urine malodorous with a "fishy" smell. Diabetic coma makes the breath smell sweet. Arsenic poisoning has a sharp and musty odour.

Children usually do not smell, but a musty odour emanates from if they are neglected and uncared for. If there is a persistent offensive smell from a child it must be investigated. It may be due to a post nasal drip, adenoids, tonsillitis, mouth breathing, caries teeth, chronic suppurative ear infection, or a foreign body (pebbles, nuts etc) inserted into a convenient orifice like the nose, ear or vagina.

A diet with excessive fat, garlic and spices consumed over a prolonged period can produce an unpleasant sharp garlicky odour.

Smoking and alcohol impart a specific odour which is present in the breath, skin and clothes of the individual.

Halitosis or simple bad breath may be due to poor oral hygiene, caries teeth or gum disease. Uncontrolled and excessive bacterial over growth in the stomach in patients with cancer can cause foul smelling breath. Severe lung infection also produces bad breath.

Normal breath contains a combination of 22 volatile alkanes, and benzene compounds. The medical profession used to rely on the characteristic odour emitted by certain diseases to reach a tentative diagnosis. Experienced brilliant clinicians sometimes diagnosed the disease en route to the bed before seeing or examining the patient.

Advances in laboratory techniques made this clinical skill unnecessary. Recently however, research is being done to develop an electronic robotic nose to smell certain diseases. The concept of an instrumental 'breathalyser' for rapid diagnosis and non-invasive screening is becoming a realistic possibility. Having lost the greater part of our olfactory senses to evolution we now have to rely on machines to perform the same function.

Hyperhidrosis (excessive sweating) is a difficult problem quite different from body odour. The two are not necessarily associated. Without bacterial action, sweat is odourless. A person with hyperhidrosis is drenched in sweat. This may occur in any part of the body but is commonest on the palms and soles. Writing may become difficult and footwear slippery. The person has to keep wiping their hands or else the paper becomes damp. It can become incapacitating. This is due to unbalanced sympathetic over activity.

Medications like the anti cholinergic group of drugs can be tried. The hands and feet can be soaked in boric powder solutions. It may eventually require surgical treatment (sympathectomy) if it is incapacitating.

Body odour can be reduced by bathing twice a day, morning and evening. This is especially required for children and working people as they return from school and office covered with dirt, dust and sweat. Use soap with trichlorhexidine and a 15 % TFA (total fatty acid) content (Dial, Neko) to reduce skin bacteria. Gently wash the skin with a scrubber or loofa . This removes the dead skin and extra sebaceous secretions.

Remove extra unwanted hair in the groin and underarm area by trimming, shaving, waxing or with epilating creams. This reduces the area retaining sweat, and hence bacterial growth and odour. It also increases the effectiveness of body sprays, antiperspirants and deodorants.

Clothes should be made from natural fibres like cotton and changed daily. Do not wear the clothes again before washing them as this produces a clinging smell of stale sweat.

Brush the teeth morning and evening. Take care of dental problems promptly.

Be conscious of your body odour. If you want to know if you smell ask your mother. She is probably the only person who will be frank enough to tell you the truth.

CHAPTER 18

HEAT AND DUST

Rising temperatures and power cuts have delivered us a double whammy. Summer has not only arrived early this year, the temperature is rising to unbearable levels. Fans, air coolers and air-conditioners should help, but they all require electricity, a scarce and rationed commodity. This is just a prelude. If the weather forecasts are to be believed , the worst is yet to come.

As the outside temperature soars to 39° and 40°C our bodies struggle to maintain an internal body temperature of 37°C. This has to remain constant come winter or summer, irrespective of the environmental temperature for our internal organs to function. Our skin with its plentiful blood supply and 2–4 million sweat glands efficiently performs this function .

If the outside temperature rises, the body starts to heat up. The brain immediately sends signals to the skin blood vessels causing them to dilate. Heat is then lost to the environment by conduction and convection. In order for this to be effective:

> ➢ The external temperature should be lower than the body temperature. Conduction and convection are not going to work when it is a sweltering 40°C outside.

> ➢ The clothes worn should be loose fitting and light coloured. Swathing the body in tight fitting dark synthetic fabrics prevents heat loss and helps the body "overheat."

> ➢ Try to stay indoors in the "heat of the day." Temperatures are cooler in the shade and in buildings.

> ➢ If you must go out use a black umbrella.

The increased blood supply is followed by sweating. Clear beads of sweat form on the skin coating it in a fine film. As this evapourates the body temperature drops. This cooling mechanism breaks down if the climate is both hot and sultry. The humidity prevents the evapouration of sweat. Adequate fluids have to be drunk for sweat to form. Hypertonic aerated fizzy drinks, glucose water, caffeinated tea and coffee or alcohol do not help. The best liquids are lightly salted buttermilk, lime juice, tender coconut water or commercially available correctly reconstituted ORS solutions.

Sweating mechanisms are poorly developed in children under the age of 4 years. They are also inefficient in the elderly, over the age of 65 years. These two extremes are more likely to suffer from the effects of heat.

If the cooling mechanism fails, painful heat cramps first occur in the larger groups of muscles like those of the leg. This can progress, if ignored, to heat illness or exhaustion manifested as weakness, dizziness, palpitations, rapid breathing and fainting. If the body temperature continues to rise to 40.6oC or higher, heat stroke can occur. The skin becomes hot and dry. Sweating mechanisms cease to function and as the high temperature effects the brain, confusion, coma and seizures can occur. Heat stroke can be fatal .

As soon as it is apparent that a person may be suffering from heat exhaustion :

- ➢ Place them in a cool shaded area.
- ➢ Remove unnecessary clothes
- ➢ Switch on the fan
- ➢ Sponge them down with tepid water
- ➢ Feed them salted fluids. Add 1 tsp (5gms) of salt to 1 litre of water

Itch and scratch, that is what summer prickly heat does to us. The red goose bumps itch intolerably and rapidly spread all over the body making the skin look like a bitter gourd. Prime time television is full of advertisements advocating "cooling" talcum powder guaranteed to make you feel like you are in the Himalayas. This is good for sales but bad for the body. Talcum powder blocks the sweat pores.

Prickly heat occurs when dirt blocks the sweat pores. The best way to tackle it is to bathe twice a day applying the soap with a terry cloth, herbal scrubber or loofah and not directly on the skin. Talcum powder aggravates the problem, as talc is actually made up of finely powdered combinations of ground zinc stearate, and silicates. When they combine with sweat they form a chalky precipitate which actually blocks skin pores . Talcum powder applied to the groin and genital areas can migrate through the vagina, uterus, and fallopian tubes to the ovary. It is carcinogenic to the lining of the ovary. The size of particles is so small that they are easily air borne. Inhaled talc can reach the smallest areas of the lung. It can then cause pneumonia or inflammation and swelling of the airways. This can be fatal in babies.

To prevent prickly heat

➤ Bathe twice a day using a bacteriocidal soap like Neko using a loofah

➤ Add a teaspoon of sodium bicarbonate to the water

➤ Wear clothes made of natural fibers like cotton which breathe and do not trap the sweat.

CHAPTER 19

PRECIOUS EYES

Eyes, their shape, colour, position, size, and symmetry, are unique and reflect personality. The steady, unfaltering, slate grey gaze of the newborn can remain unchanged throughout life or become the shifty-eyed look of the habitual criminal.

The colour of the eyes is inherited. It varies according to the amount of pigment present in the eyeball or iris. The colour of the adult eye is established by the age of one year. If there is no pigment at all, the eyes are blue. If the iris has a great deal of pigment it is black. Sometimes the two eyes can be of different colours. Although this is a minor abnormality which may be isolated, it warrants a search for other internal malformations. As a person grows older, fine new blood vessels can grow across the iris turning it pinkish red in diabetics or those with ischemic heart disease.

The distance between the two eyes may be increased (hyperteleorism), or be less than normal when the eyes are "close set". Both may be familial and normal. It does however warrant a search for other associated abnormalities. The slant of the eyes is measured by drawing an imaginary line connecting the two ends of the eyes. It is normally either straight or slightly upward (Mongoloid). If it is downwards (anti- Mongoloid) then again other internal organ abnormalities should be searched for.

Skin folds present near the nose, called epicanthic folds make the eyes appear "Chinese". This is normal in some families and races. In others, it may be associated with Down's syndrome (Mongolism) or congenital heart disease. It is a genetic marker and warrants a careful search for other abnormalities.

Ptosis is a condition where there is drooping of one or more eyelids. Congenital ptosis causes a peculiar upward gaze with a tilted neck as the child attempts to see through the droopy lid. It can usually be surgically corrected. It can occur bilaterally in adults in diseases which cause muscle weakness like myasthenia gravis.

If one eye is smaller than the other, it may be due to innocuous facial asymmetry present from birth. Retention of fluid in the body as a result of renal or cardiac disease can cause bilateral eyelid swelling and a puffy appearance. In hyperthyroidism or as a result of a tumour in the orbit of the eye, one eye may appear to bulge out.

Sometimes eyes exhibit constant rapid side to side movement with a shifty wavering gaze. This condition, called nystagmus, may be inherited and familial. The vision itself can be normal. Secondary nystagmus can appear after childhood due to disease processes either in the vestibular apparatus of the ear or in the central nervous system.

The eyelids may sometimes be infected with bacteria forming "styes." Eyelashes can be infected and sticky. Infestation of the eyes can occur with head lice as well. Gentle cleansing twice a day with a non-irritating baby shampoo is curative and painless.

Beautiful almond-shaped eyes have their appeal enhanced by outlining them with kajal, kohl and eyeliner. But, sometimes these products contain chemicals that can cause allergic reactions and can be dangerous. Application to the eyes of children is not advisable.

The eyes may sometimes appear red in colour, or itch. If there is a clear watery discharge and tearing, it is probably due to an allergy or a viral infection. A more purulent discharge is probably due to bacterial conjunctivitis and may require antibiotic drops. Worm infestation and tuberculosis can cause a characteristic red reaction with a central white nodule. Blood shot eyes are not necessarily the sign of alcoholism. It can be due to a sudden haemorrhage into the sclera as a result of a severe cough. Vitamin A deficiency causes silvery scales to form in the outer angles of the eyes.

Cataracts can develop with age, with excessive exposure of unprotected eyes (without sunglasses) to sunlight and harsh weather conditions or with metabolic disorders like diabetes. They can be unilateral or bilateral, partial or complete. Cataracts can occur in children. Usually in such cases they can be inherited, or be a part of certain syndromes, or occur as a result of congenital rubella or toxoplasmosis infection.

The eyes of comatose patients should be taped shut and lubricated with artificial tears to prevent corneal damage and loss of eyesight.

A complete eye check up should be done every year.

It involves :

➤ A test of vision using a computer or having the person read jumbled alphabets or symbols using one eye at a time from eye charts placed at a fixed distance.

➤ An evaluation of the visual field is needed. Sometimes there can be a constriction of the visual field in the centre or a loss of vision in the periphery. Both these are ominous signs and may be due to a tumour in the brain.

➤ A fundoscopy with an ophthalmoscope should be done to evaluate the retina. Changes due to diabetes, hypertension and arteriosclerosis, can be seen and reflect vessel changes elsewhere in the body. Characteristic diagnostic deposits can be seen in the eye in diseases like tuberculosis and toxoplasmosis.

➤ The pressure in the eye should be measured. Increased pressure is called glaucoma. It can be medically and surgically treated. Untreated glaucoma is one of the commonest causes of acquired blindness.

➤ A slit lamp examination of the cornea should be done to pick up abnormalities.

Defective vision can be corrected with spectacles, contact lenses and laser surgery. Cataract removal now involves high tech placement of artificial lenses in the eye itself making post surgery vision almost normal. The surgical procedure itself takes only a few minutes and is usually very successful.

Sight is precious. Donate your eyes after you die. Register today for eye donation. Let someone else see with your eyes when you no longer need them.

Chapter 20

Deafness and Hearing Loss

"What did you say?"

The boy stood helplessly as his classmates shouted, "retard, deaf, idiot". The meaningless words made jumbled sounds in his head. He stared silently and angrily as he was unable to respond. Children can be very cruel. It is easy to torment some one who cannot hear or retort appropriately.

Hearing loss affects 10% of the young adult population, and 35% of those over 65 years. It may be complete or partial. It may affect sounds of only a certain pitch.

However, the boy in the story was not really deaf or retarded. All he had was a defect in the area of the brain that processes the sounds heard. This results in faulty interpretation. Anything spoken, though clearly heard, became a meaningless jumble in his brain. This can be an isolated defect or associated with other learning disabilities like dyslexia or hyperactive attention deficit disorder. School performance is poor and the child tends to "fail".

Normal life is affected by impaired hearing. To live safely in society we need all our higher senses, sound, sight and speech.

Deaf children have poor attention spans, and an inability to comprehend. This results in sub optimal school performance. If the defect is not recognized, they are punished harshly for "not listening, obeying or understanding". They are frustrated and unable to cope with the academic requirements. The school drop out rate is high.

Deaf adults are accident-prone, isolated, lonely and sidelined in society. Those with noise induced hearing loss suffer from stress, irritability, poor concentration and depression. Unless subtitles are available they are unable to entertain themselves watching movies or television.

Hearing loss may be acute or chronic, complete or partial, congenital or acquired.

In 0.5–1%children the cause of hearing loss is genetic. It is usually due to inheritance of an autosomal dominant gene. There are many deaf members in the same family. The abnormal gene appears regularly and in every generation. The autosomal recessive forms are more difficult to diagnose. Two abnormal genes have to be inherited, one from each parent, for the patient to become deaf. Many generations have to be screened to find affected individuals and establish a genetic pattern. Consanguineous marriages increase the chances of the child inheriting deafness as recessive genes may be inherited from both parents and then expressed.

Deafness may be suspected if the ear is anatomically abnormal. There may be hereditary malformations like the absence of a patent ear canal, or the ear may be smaller and of a different shape.

The ears can be damaged before birth if the mother has infections like toxoplasmosis, herpes or congenital rubella during the first trimester of pregnancy. These children are deaf. The defect is isolated and does not run in families. This can be prevented by:

➤ Avoiding exposure to cats during pregnancy to prevent toxoplasmosis.

➤ Prior immunization with the MMR (measles mumps and rubella) vaccine to prevent rubella infection.

➤ Genital herpes is a sexually transmitted disease. Prevention is entirely in the hands of the individual by avoiding exposure to multiple partners. Condoms, if correctly used reduce the incidence of herpes.

Deafness can occur during the process of birth, if the child born is premature, asphyxiated, small (less than 1.5 kg) or the develops a severe infection (septicaemia). Infection usually occurs during passage through the birth canal. All these conditions can be prevented with the improved reproductive and antenatal care.

Children frequently develop ear infections. This is because the connection between the throat and the ear (Eustachian tube) is straighter in children. It can be blocked by food and milk, which accidentally enters as a result of faulty positioning while feeding. While feeding, the head should ideally be cradled in the mother's arms at an angle of 45 degrees. Children who can sit should be seated in a rocker or a high chair.

Many mothers force feed uncooperative, struggling and reluctant children placing them in the supine (lying down) position pinning them down on the floor or on their legs. Bottle feeds, or force-feeding in the lying down position, is dangerous, ineffective and unnecessary. Food and liquids can enter the Eustachian tube and then the middle ear leading to secondary infection.

People disembark from aircraft with earaches, giddiness, partial deafness and head aches. The pain is often intolerable, and the giddiness leads to loss of balance. Sometimes a watery discharge oozes from one ear. This is not the best or most enjoyable way to start a well earned holiday. The rapid difference in pressure during ascent and descent produces an imbalance in the middle ear called "barotitis media" which results in pain.

Any ear infection should be promptly and adequately treated. The doctor's instructions regarding dosage and duration of medication should be strictly followed. Concomitant use of saline nose drops and steam inhalation relieves blockage of the nose and facilitates drainage of secretions. Initial infection, inadequately treated, results in a chronically discharging or permanently blocked "glue" ear.

A patent ear canal may be blocked by skin and debris, or with a build up of naturally occurring wax. This prevents conduction of sounds to brain and produces hearing difficulties and pain.

Some commonly used antibiotics like streptomycin, kannamicin and gentamicin are toxic to the ear.

Infections like meningitis, encephalitis and abscesses, or brain tumours can cause hearing impairment. Ear infection if left untreated can lead to meningitis as the ear is very close to the brain.

Noise pollution, especially in urban areas increases the chances of eventual hearing impairment. Airport workers, truck drivers and disc jockeys are exposed to 90–100 decibels of noise continuously. Firecrackers, rock concerts and banned cone loudspeakers are used during political rallies emit sound at the intensity of approximately140 decibels. Regular prolonged exposure eventually results in perceptible hearing loss.

Personal stereo players, which play music directly into the ear with earphones, are a newer cause of hearing impairment. The volume should be carefully adjusted to the minimum BEFORE the earphones are inserted and the system switched on not after the plugs are inserted into the ear.

Hearing loss called "prebycusis" may occur spontaneously and naturally with aging. It tends to run in families and is aggravated by smoking. It may be part of menieres disease if it is associated with giddiness and "ringing" in the ears.

Place your fore fingers in each ear so that all sounds are blocked. Make a rhythmic ooh sound while breathing out for 1 minute. This is a simple yogic exercise to preserve hearing and prevent age related hearing loss.

Evaluation of hearing loss should be done early and corrective measures taken. Hearing aids are available for all age groups. Surgical procedures to correct defects and hi tech inner ear implants are now available and can be inserted.

Hearing impaired people can be taught to lip read. Visual clues and subtitles to supplement vocal instructions can make life easier for them

As a society we should not encourage loud "bombs" and other firecrackers during the festival season. Silent aesthetically pleasing firework displays are a safer option.

Protect your ears and those of your children with cotton balls or earmuffs if you feel they are going to be exposed to loud noises.

Try to conserve the hearing you have. Treat the handicapped with kindness. Remember as age advances you too may develop a hearing disability and be the butt of cruel pranks and unkind jokes.

Chapter 21

Breasts, Development, Changes and Disease

Many teenagers (boys and girls) have walked into my clinic over the last three decades, worried about their breasts. The girls are upset because the breasts are too big or small, begin to appear too early or too late, or are asymmetric. The boys are troubled because breasts have appeared at all!

Breasts have fascinated human beings of all ages. It starts at birth with the baby automatically "rooting" for the mother's nipple and sucking hungrily. Then toddlers are spellbound by the fact that some mothers have "ready to drink" pre sterilized feeding bottles permanently fixed to their chest, while others buy plastic feeding bottles in shops. Later in adult life, symmetric globular breasts are associated with a perfect figure and potential for the Miss Universe title.

With the newer plastic and cosmetic surgery techniques, any adult can have perfect breasts. The size and shape can be altered with cosmetic surgery and silicone implants to produce the desired result.

Babies can develop enlarged breasts soon after birth. It can occur in male and female children. This is due to exposure to the mothers hormones while in the uterus. It subsides spontaneously provided it is left untouched. Massaging and manipulation gives rise to secondary bacterial infection and abscess formation.

Breasts develop during adolescence between the ages of 9 and 13. A bud like tender swelling may appear first on one side many months before actual breast development. This might worry the parents and the child, especially as sometimes these breast buds are very tender.

Half of adolescent boys can develop breasts. This condition called gynaecomastia and is due a temporary hormonal imbalance. It usually disappears spontaneously in 6–18 months. If it persists, investigations and treatment are required for correctable causes. Cosmetic surgery may eventually be required.

The sudden appearance of gynaecomastia in an adult male requires evaluation. It is due to oestrogen excess and hormonal imbalance. This can occur with certain medications, alcohol consumption, cannabis, other recreational drugs or a hormone producing tumour.

Breast cancer is a common cause of cancer in women. The risk of developing breast cancer increased with:

➢ Advancing age

➢ A family history of female relatives with cancer of the breast or ovary. This is because some genes like the BRAC1 and 2 are associated with these cancers. 10% of young women with breast cancer carry this gene. This genetic predisposition causes the cancer to occur before the age of 40, in multiple relatives, and in one or both breasts.

➢ Long exposure of the breasts to hormones, with an early onset of menstruation (before 12) and late menopause (after 55) increases the risk of cancer.

➢ Threatened abortion was earlier treated with diethylstilbestrol (DES): This medicine is associated with an increased risk of developing breast cancer.

➢ Hormone replacement therapy increases the risk of developing breast cancer if it is continued for many years after menopause.

➢ Having no children at all or conceiving the first child after the age of 30 increases the risk.

➢ Multiple pregnancies decrease the risk.

Breast feeding decreases the risk.

Women should be "breast aware" as early detection of breast cancer increases the chance of successful treatment and long term survival. Knowledge about the changes and feel of your own breasts at different times of your menstrual cycle will help in early detection of any change.

A breast self examination should be done at the same time each month preferably just after menstruation.

- ➢ Lie down on the floor
- ➢ Use the sensitive pads of the middle three fingers of the left hand to examine the right breast. Use the right hand for the left breast.
- ➢ Use a circular, wedge and then a vertical motion to feel every part of the breast including the tip extending into the armpit.
- ➢ Look at the skin of the breasts in the mirror.
- ➢ Check the appearance of the nipple.

Lumps appear in the breast at various stages in a woman's life. 90% of these lumps are either fluid filled cysts or a harmless non cancerous overgrowth of fibrous and glandular tissue. These are called fibrocystic disease of the breast or fibroadenosis.

Sometimes the hormonal changes associated with normal menstruation will make breasts appear painful, lumpy and engorged in the 7–10 days prior to the onset of bleeding. All these are normal.

Danger signs are:

- ➢ A sudden change in the size or shape of the breasts
- ➢ Dimpling of the skin so that it looks like an orange peel
- ➢ Palpable lumps
- ➢ Inversion of the nipple
- ➢ A bloodstained discharge from nipple
- ➢ A rash on or around the nipple
- ➢ A swelling in the armpit or neck.

A doctor should be immediately consulted if any of the above are found or suspected.

An evaluation of a suspicious breast requires a physical examination, an ultrasound, a mammogram an MRI scan and an FNAC (fine needle aspiration cytology). Sometimes a removal of the mass or a biopsy may be required.

Summary dismissal of the symptoms of an anxious woman, or a reassurance that the lump will go away without the above investigations is dangerous. Cancer can be a great deceiver. It can occur at any age and in any person. Males are not exempt.

Mammograms are ideally done for all women over the age of 50 every 2–3 years. It involves only a small dose of radiation and picks up small lumps which cannot be felt manually. It is expensive and sometimes ultrasound scanning is used instead.

Breast cancer is easily detectable, treatable and curable. All it takes is three minutes of your time to check your breasts every month.

CHAPTER 22

HIV/AIDS

Living in a fool's paradise

"It cannot happen to me! AIDS occurs in commercial sex workers (CSW), IV drug users, the uneducated and the socio- economically under privileged." How often we have heard these words! They are a misnomer, and nothing could be further from the truth.

India has been voted the 2nd sexiest nation, only 0.4% behind Brazil. Yet our prevalence of AIDS is 0.5%, just behind Africa, while in Brazil it is 0.1%. Our stone sculptures and carvings are mute testimony to our traditional cultural obsession with sex. No amount of legislation can change that. Banning public displays of affection and targeting the commercial sex trade will not help. It will only drive the activity further underground. Realization, awareness and change has to come from within, with knowledge and education.

Our cultural heritage, family values or wealth cannot prevent HIV infection if we indulge in sex with multiple partners, whether they are sex workers, co-workers, friends or relatives. "Another woman" or "another man" becomes a third party in an equation, that, for health reasons, should involve only two consenting sexually faithful adults.

HIV infection can occur in any one with a single episode of unprotected intercourse. An asymptomatic infected person, while apparently healthy, can pass on the disease to others, through contact with blood, semen, vaginal secretions or breast milk. Unfortunately, mentally, as a nation we suffer delusions about "decent" women and men and consider sex outside marriage with them safe. Anyone, even someone apparently healthy can carry the HIV virus. Once a third partner is introduced into a relationship sexual acts are Russian roulette. Condoms, if used regularly, though protective, are not magic bullets, as leakage has been known to occur.

In the press and in the minds of people, the terms HIV and AIDS are incorrectly interchanged. HIV is a virus, which enters the body and causes an initial infection which may be asymptomatic, or produce only mild flu like symptoms with tiredness, aches and pains, sore throat and lethargy. This may last up to a month and then there may be apparent total recovery. The HIV can then remain dormant for 10–15 years. It then replicates and multiplies in the infected person, causing deterioration in the body's ability to fight other infections. Some of these infections may have already been present subclincally in the body, suppressed by inherent natural immunity. Simple infections like tuberculosis and fungal infections become uncontrolled and rampant. The compromised body is unable to cope with even the mildest of infections. This can eventually result in full-blown AIDS and death if left untreated.

Sometimes tumours and cancers are the first signs that the person is immunocopromised. Initial diagnosis of HIV infection therefore depends on a high degree of suspicion on the part of the treating physician.

In India between the incidence of HIV infection is apparently highest in the states of Gujarat., Goa , Pondicherry, Maharashtra, Tamil Nadu and Manipur. These statistics are obtained from tests done on women attending antenatal clinics and from STD (sexually transmitted disease) clinics.

The fallacy is that in many districts, structured antenatal care and STD testing is lacking or not utilized. Many women (even educated ones) object to the HIV test as part of their routine antenatal care. "Sex diseases" are undocumented, improperly diagnosed and confirmatory tests are not done. Medication is unethically dispensed in suppressive non-therapeutic doses by unqualified quacks. Hence the exact numbers of infected persons is not known and numbers are only projected or assumed.

The ratio of the CSW to client is higher in India (less workers/ more clients) than in other countries. There is no legalized prostitution, registration, compulsory condom use or mandatory testing of sex workers. These numbers also are not known with certainty. They are a migrant group and some work part time. As they indulge in sex with other multiple partners, they acquire other sexually transmitted infections. These infections are dangerous in themselves. They also increase susceptibility to the HIV virus.

People are on the move. A large migrant population reaches the cities seeking work. They leave their spouses behind. Many indulge in high risk behaviour. They may become HIV positive. They return home to other geographical areas once a year and eventually spouses in their home towns in are infected.

There has also been an explosive increase in the numbers of IV drug abusers. They also visit commercial sex workers. They become HIV positive within a year.

HIV transmission does not always occur from CSW through heterosexual sex.

Indian surveys have shown that male-to-male sex (MSM) does occur. 17% of Indian males have engaged in MSM. Some are coerced, others raped, many are willing participants. Of these men, 52% also have sex with women, either with female CSW, or as 42% are married, to unsuspecting wives. Incestuous MSM often occurs within the family, between cousins, uncles and nephews or distant older relatives. Sometimes, teachers or neighbours are involved. The acts are secretive and the perpetuator and victim maintain silence, out of a sense of fear, shame or outrage. Condoms are not used during these encounters. The male involved may be a married bisexual with children.

In our global village, with affordable travel, package tours and multinational businesses, both men and women engage in sex with unknown or multiple partners in the secluded anonymity of hotel rooms in other countries and regions. In SE Asia, a favourite tourist destination, 7.1 million persons (1/5 of the total HIV cases in the world) are infected. Indians are not exempt. With affordable travel and freely available foreign exchange, many upwardly mobile Indians and visit these areas.

"Sex" is still a taboo three-letter word in Indian society.

Children do not receive much sex education at the school level when they need it. There are widely expressed fears that knowledge will only make teenagers more promiscuous. Yet, statistics show that 5–20 % of the 15– 50-year-old male population visit sex workers. 3% of the females in the same age group admit to premarital sex.

Ignorance places our young populations at risk as they may impulsively indulge in risky promiscuous behaviour without adequate protective information.

Fear and social stigma attached to the disease makes reaching proper testing facilities a delayed fly by night operation. To overcome this, the government has now provided several "VCTC" (voluntary counselling and testing centres) centres, where anonymous free testing and counselling are offered.

A rapid test for HIV (ELISA) can give a false positive reaction, especially in persons who have recently had malaria or dengue (both present in India). It should therefore be reconfirmed. A second ELISA can be done, or the more expensive confirmatory western blot test.

A HIV "positive" test result is no longer a death sentence. The lifesaving HAART (highly active anti retroviral therapy) can suppress the infection, improve the immune status, prevent lethal opportunistic infections and enable the person to lead a reasonably productive life. Medication is life long, with no drug holidays. There are some accompanying dietary restrictions and a few unpleasant side effects.

HAART drugs were prohibitively expensive. Availability of generic drugs have changed this scenario. Indian drug companies have taken the initiative to provide generic HAART. The government, NGOs, philanthropic drug companies, now provide HAART at the reasonable cost of Rs1000–1500 per month.

If you are afraid that you have contracted HIV or a STD :

➢ Seek help from qualified personnel or visit the nearest VCTC.

➢ Doctors are bound legally and by oath to secrecy. They cannot divulge your medical condition to anyone.

> ➤ Panic and delay in seeking medical help will make the disease progress not disappear.
>
> ➤ Avoid quacks, miracle cures, and untried, unproven, unscientific, natural and herbal remedies.

IEC (Information, education and communication) holds the key to tackling this emerging menacing problem. It helps youngsters to resist peer pressure and make informed choices about safe behaviour and lifestyle.

Knowledge prolongs life, while ignorance leads to death.

CHAPTER 23

PICA, — PERVERTED APPETITE

The two year old seated herself in front of the flowerpot, dug her fingers into the soft brown mud and proceeded to stuff it into her mouth. It was a disgusting sight, bystanders stared, and the embarrassed mother commented, "I wish she would eat her meals with as much enthusiasm."

Perverted appetite with a desire to eat items not generally considered "food" is called Pica. The word is derived from the Latin name for "magpie" a bird notorious for its lack of dietary discretion. Magpies eat anything and everything, but they have tough intestines which somehow digest or eliminate articles eaten. Human beings do not have intestines like that of the magpie. We have to exert dietary discretion as we cannot digest articles that do not belong to the food chain.

Pica is an international phenomenon affecting people of all ages and both sexes. It tends to be more common in the underprivileged, uneducated, mentally challenged and psychologically handicapped. It is aggravated by lack of supervision from an authority figure.

In some areas, pica is culturally accepted, with consumption of clay and chalk believed to be medicinal and protective against diseases like jaundice, diarrhoea and morning sickness. Sometimes, it is believed to confer mystical powers, especially if eaten at auspicious times like during the full moon nights.

Pregnancy has long been associated with perverted appetites and craving, which unfortunately is so accepted as part of the norm that they are ignored by patients and family members.

Pica has to be differentiated from bullemia nervosa, which is characterized by periodic intervals of binge eating. Unusually large amount of a particular food item are consumed, with the feeling that the eating is out of control. The difference is that edible food items are consumed, whereas in pica non-edible non-food items are eaten.

Items consumed by affected individuals include dirt, clay, raw rice, slate and slate pencils, paint, plaster, chalk, coffee grounds, cigarette ashes, cigarette butts, burnt match heads, rust, glue, hair, buttons, paper, sand, toothpaste, soap, sea shells, and broken crockery.

Children lack subtlety and openly exhibit their strange food preferences. They tend to explore their environment. The oral cavity is one of the most sensitive areas of the body, and one of the ways to determine the consistency of an object is to put it into the mouth. This stage of oral fixation is usually outgrown by the age of two, but if it persists it eventually metamorphosis into adult pica.

Pica requires treatment and is out of control and when there is repetitive consumption of the non-food item for a month or longer after the age of two in a mentally normal individual with an inability to rationally control the behaviour.

Embarrassed adults hide their pica and do not mention it during visits to the physician. They fail to understand the significance of the problem, and do not realize that it is medical. They and feel guilt and shame about their actions.

There are many theories about the cause of pica, with it related to nutritional deficiencies, sensory stimulation, and physiologic and psychosocial deprivation.

So far no specific biological or biochemical abnormality has been proved to cause this aberration.

Nutritional deficiency of iron, zinc or calcium may trigger appetite regulating brain enzymes and specific cravings. The non-food items consumed in an effort to assuage this do not supply the deficient minerals, and the person is caught in a vicious cycle. The more they eat, the more they crave.

Geophagia (eating clay and mud) may be habit like having a cigarette in the morning. It may be an acquired behavioural response to unexpressed stress. It in itself can cause iron deficiency aggravating the problem further.

Emotional disturbances causing pica are more difficult to tackle, especially if the person is autistic, mentally challenged or has a psychiatric illness. Corporal punishment and ridicule only aggravates pica further, and is eventually self defeating.

Pica is not just a social embarrassment; it can be dangerous to health. Hair and chalk can form an indigestible solid mass in the stomach resulting in an intestinal block, which has to be surgically tackled. Mud contains eggs of parasitic worms predisposing the individual to heavy infestation. Some chemicals consumed are toxic potentially harmful substances, such as those contaminated by heavy metals like lead or mercury. It can result in lead and mercury poisoning. Toothpaste damages intestinal villi. It has been implicated in some of the malabsorption syndromes. Even crunching ice and refrigerator frost damages teeth enamel!

Although mature individuals may deny their unusual cravings to their doctor, they may exhibit other symptoms like fatigue, palpitations, light-headedness, and shortness of breath. These may be accompanied by signs of iron and vitamin deficiency, like pallor, thinned out spooned concave nails, flattened tongue papillae, superficial erosions in the mucosa of the mouth and fissuring at the angles of the lips.

Even though the cause is unproven, treatment is successful. Pica responds dramatically to iron, zinc, multivitamin and calcium supplements supported by deworming.

While administering these nutritional supplements, for them to be optimally absorbed, certain principles have to be kept in mind. Zinc and iron compete for the same absorption sites in the intestine. They cannot be administered together as they "lock" the absorption site, and both are eventually not absorbed but eliminated. They need to be given separately on different days. Calcium precipitates with iron and zinc and prevents its absorption. It should be given separately 12 hours apart. Manufacturers forget these principles and recommend administration of a "hotchpotch" of irrational formulations to patients, usually an elixir, tonic or capsule containing iron, zinc, calcium, vitamins and trace elements all mixed together.

After a sufficient and satisfactory response to pica, no further treatment is required. However a close watch, for recurrence of the symptoms, may have to kept on the individual, for a couple of months, by an involved and motivated caregiver.

CHAPTER 24

MOSQUITOES

Help! Airborne mosquito attack!

The "enemy" air force strikes at dusk and dawn in times of war. In India we are similarly affected, as we face hordes of attacking "haemophagous" (blood sucking) mosquitoes at twilight. We strive to keep disease bearing Aedes, Anopheles and Culex mosquitoes out of our homes and away from our skin. Some have been are aptly christened by entomologists with expressive scientific names like "Aedes vexans", "Aedes excrucians", and "Coquillettidia perturbans", which match their behaviour and reputations!

Mosquitoes survive as they are hardy and adapt to a changing environment. Their reproduction is rapid, prolific and efficient. The fertilized female requires a blood meal (preferably human) before laying eggs. The transmission of the disease-causing organisms from one person to another occurs during this feeding process.

Mating occurs at dawn and dusk, and it is at this time, when the fertilized female searches for a blood meal, that human attacks are at their peak. Gravid female mosquitoes, of all species, after their mandatory blood meal are able to fly up to two km in search of stagnant, brackish or slowly flowing water to lay their eggs. (Not many pregnant women can run for a distance of two km to deliver!) The quantity of water needed is very small. Even the few ml in an upturned bottle cap is sufficient. If all the stages of the life cycle are completed successfully in 10 days a new generation has taken over from the old.

Mosquitoes are dangerous as their bite spreads diseases. India is endemic for malaria, filarial, dengue and encephalitis spread by mosquitoes. We have not been able to eradicate any of these, and now even "control" is slipping away.

India and many other tropical countries have been endemic for malaria for centuries. Even today, despite our urban high tech lifestyle, we are no closer to eradicating the disease

After living for generations in close association with the malarial parasite, the local population has developed adaptive mechanisms and a certain amount of resistance. Some of our genetic traits confer some immunity to malaria, proving the age-old supposition that "only the strong survive."

Malaria was present during the crusades and was partially responsible for chronic ill- health and debility in the soldiers and their commandants, leading to the eventual fizzling out of the wars. The same physicians treated soldiers belonging to both the Muslim and Christian armies with extracts of the cinchona bark. We, today, still use purified quinine compounds from the same source. This does not speak well for the state of research into medications for the treatment of malaria.

Many of the British developed malaria when they colonized India. They gravitated to Gymkhana clubs and consumed "gin and tonic". The bitter tonic water contained quinine, (the original cinchona bark product) and the gin made it palatable. The regular tipplers received a certain amount of protection against malaria.

In the first half of the twentieth century, 30 % of the Tennessee valley population developed malaria. The US government swung into action, swamps were drained and treated, research done, new drugs developed and the disease eradicated in the USA.

Now, the people living in non- tropical areas get infected very rarely. The mosquito can, however be transported accidentally in an airplane. In this way, sometimes, the infection may be brought to a non-tropical country. Also infected returning travellers can rarely bring the disease with them.

The developed nations have therefore lost interest in a disease that does not directly affect them. No new drugs have been developed in the last 20 years; the mosquito and the malarial parasite are becoming increasingly resistant to currently used pesticides and medications.

SARS eventually killed 973 people. The US government spent 3.2 billion dollars investigating and evaluating the outbreak. In contrast, there are 300 million cases of malaria a year, and 1–2 million of these are fatal. Yet, less than 0.5 million is spend globally on malaria research.

Africa is in the same situation as India. Moved by the plight of thousands of unfortunate children who die of malaria in these two countries, the Gates foundation has recently invested $250 million in malaria research. They are hoping to change this scenario and develop preventive vaccines and newer techniques and medications to control this age old disease.

Typical malaria occurs in non-immune individuals. After a variable incubation period, it presents as fever, headache, aches, pains and diarrhoea. The typical high fever occurring every third or alternate day with shivering and sweats takes longer to establish itself. The disease may also creep on insidiously eventually cause economically devastating anaemia, fatigue and lethargy. It is particularly severe and dangerous in children, pregnant women and in people who do not have a functioning spleen.

Malaria strikes susceptible individuals 9 to 14 days after the initial mosquito bite. The flu like symptoms progress rapidly as the parasite invades the blood stream destroying blood cells on its way to various organs in the body. The symptoms produced depend on the targeted organ. In the brain it causes fatal cerebral malaria

The diagnosis of malaria is based on the examination of blood smears. Once confirmed, a complete course of therapy should be given. This is because the parasite can remain dormant in the liver, only to re-emerge after a variable period and cause a relapsing or chronic infection.

Treatment usually entails a 3-day course of chloroquin followed by a 2 or 3 week course of primaquin. Unfortunately ignorance often makes patients discontinue the therapy once they "feel better", keeping some tablets for later use. Sometimes, unqualified individuals randomly dispense an "antimalarial" along with paracemetol and single dose of an antibiotic for "fever". This irrational therapy may be successful, as both a bacterial infection and malaria may be suppressed. Eventually there will be a recrudescence of both diseases with a confused clinical picture confounding the treating physician.

Prevention of malaria is a better and safer than treatment of the disease.

Travellers to an endemic region need to take medical prophylaxis. This should be started before reaching the tropical country. Residents leaving the tropics rapidly loose their immunity. After residing elsewhere for a few years they are as susceptible to malaria as tourists.

Filaria is another mosquito borne disease caused by the filarial worm and carried by the culex species of mosquito. It can cause disfiguring elephantiasis with one limb enlarged disproportionately. It may affect the arm, leg or scrotum in men. This is due to blockage of the lymphatic drainage by the filarial parasite.

Dengue fever is spread by the Aedes mosquito. It varies in severity from a mild febrile illness lasting a few days to a fatal illness characterized by shock and haemorrhage.

Encephalitis or brain fever has a high mortality and is transmitted by mosquito bites.

In addition mosquito bites can be itchy and irritating, and if scratched, are prone to develop secondary bacterial infection with attendant complications.

One of the ways to tackle these diseases is to prevent breeding of the mosquitoes as far as possible.

The hardy eggs survive for long periods in dry mud or on the sides of containers, only to hatch again when water is available. Only with elimination of breeding grounds can the mosquito population be controlled.

> ➤ As you walk, turn over any empty container particularly bottles caps and coconut shells so that rainwater does not

stagnate inside. Straighten sagging canvas and plastic coverings periodically.

➢ Empty air conditioning and cooler trays. Alternatively put handful p of salt into the tray so that mosquitoes cannot breed.

➢ Do not place trays under potted plants. Empty pots and vases regularly.

➢ Fix mosquito mesh on open tanks wells and outlets.

➢ The environment around residences should be kept free from stagnant water or open drainage. If this is impossible, a fist full of rock salt or 100 ml of kerosene added to the water daily, prevents the mosquito larvae from breathing. and eventually reduces the insect population.

➢ Water used in room coolers also allows mosquitoes to breed and should be similarly treated.

➢ There are some hardy mosquito larva eating ornamental fish, Gabusia and Poecili (guppy). They are available from the municipality, malaria control program offices and in pet shops. They can be added by motivated individuals to public ponds canals and sewers.

➢ Windows and doors can be "mosquito proofed" using inexpensive plastic mesh.

➢ Sleeping inside a mosquito net is a time-tested method of preventing bites. Newer mosquito repellent impregnated nets are available.

➢ Wear full-sleeved shirts, and long pants, and cover the feet fully at dawn and dusk to prevent bites.

➢ Mosquito repellents especially ones containing lemon grass oil are fairly efficient. It is better to apply it to clothes rather than directly on the skin. They should not be applied in children less than a year old or to pregnant women.

➢ Coils, liquid repellents and mosquito mats are better avoided. They should be used in places where there are children below the age of 6 months. They can cause respiratory allergy, and lead to wheezing and sneezing in susceptible individuals.

> ➤ BTI (bacillus thuringiensis israelensis), is a naturally occurring bacterium that kills immature mosquito larvae. It is available with the government malaria control division. The substance is nontoxic to humans and can be dumped in stagnant brackish or slowly flowing water.

Many mosquitoes are now resistant to DDT and other commonly used insecticides so that they survive and reproduce despite regular spraying by government and private agencies. Spraying of the environment with insecticides causes the development of "pesticide resistance" in mosquitoes and respiratory allergies in susceptible individuals. It is eventually counterproductive.

As Indians, we should use our civic sense and work together towards the eradication of mosquitoes and malaria.

Shortsighted malaria and mosquito eradication policies based on personal financial gain rather than the common good of the nation will eventually be counterproductive and detrimental to our health and that of the generations that follow.

In our country, with plentiful human resources, and limited finances we can tackle our mosquito problem. We have to march towards this common goal together, united as a nation. After all, collectively we drove out the British. Surely we can succeed with a few mosquitoes!

CHAPTER 25

CARE OF THE HAIR—OUR CROWNING GLORY

The classical Indian beauty in paintings is depicted with limpid lotus shaped kajal lined eyes and flowing black tresses. The accompanying male figures have their "crowning glory" covered with a turban or some other device, leaving the actual quantity of hair to the imagination! Maybe it is because as a nation, genetically for generations, we have had "male pattern baldness," which is better concealed than revealed.

This typical appearance is changing now. Women are cropping their hair short and bald men with uncovered heads are visible everywhere. The characters on TV, both male and female, in advertisements, movies and serials have full heads of hair, but how much is real? Much of what we see may be extensions, attachments, hairpieces, wigs or simply computer-modified images.

If bus hoardings and advertisements are to be believed, there is a huge market for products preventing hair loss, as, all over the country, men women and children are loosing their hair.

Hair growth and loss has its own cycles, with a growing phase that lasts between two and six years, followed by a resting phase that lasts two to three months. At any given time 10% of the hair is resting and 80–90 % growing. At the end of its resting stage, the hair is shed. A loss of 75–100 hairs a day is normal. After shedding, a new hair grows from the same follicle and replaces it, starting the cycle again. Scalp hair grows about one-half inches a month. As people age, their rate of hair growth slows and the total number of hair follicles also shows a gradual decline.

If the hair loss is greater than 150 hairs per day, then there is a pathological process affecting the normal hair renewal process, which needs medical evaluation.

Remember, the effected person alone may be sensitive to his or her own hair loss, as much as 50 % of all the available hair needs to fall before it becomes obvious to the doctor.

Hair may be normally lost excessively by traction in hairstyles with the hair pulled back with clips or braided too tightly.

Hair loss may be may be due to an unnatural process of "hair pulling" called "trichotillomania" where people, particularly children, will twist and pull out their own hair, eyebrows, or lashes. It is a bad habit precipitated by psychological and social stress. There is spontaneous improvement when the harmful effects of the habit are explained and the stress factors removed. If it does not resolve, then consultation with a psychiatrist is needed.

Hair loss may be due to dietary factors with sub clinical malnutrition as a result of fad diets or crash diets, with an accompanying deficiency of proteins, vitamins and minerals.

Hormonal imbalances cause increased hair loss, with remaining hair becoming thin, brittle and lack lustre in appearance. Thyroid hormones and an abnormal alteration in the ratio between estrogens, progesterone and androgens are notorious for this. The hormonal balance can go awry during periods of stress, or during menarche, pregnancy, lactation and menopause.

The predisposition to loose hair after a certain age is genetically transmitted in families, through the mother. All the effected male members of that particular family tend to look identical when their heads are viewed from behind.

Androgens (male hormones) cause male pattern baldness. If a women has excess androgens for any reason she tends to loose her hair and become bald.

Expert evaluation is required to rule out conditions like "alopecia areata" (patchy baldness) when well-defined, circular, hairless patches are found in various areas of the scalp. Local treatment with triamcinolone or systemic treatment with finastride (in males) can initially reverse the process. One it progressed to "alopecia totalis "(loss of all the hair) treatment is not very successful.

It is heartening to know that hair loss, due to chemotherapy in cancer patients, reverses spontaneously when the treatment is discontinued.

Radiation injury and surgical scars cause permanent hair loss in the affected area

In the absence of non-reversible conditions, even if "baldness genes" are present, certain principles can be followed to preserve existing hair, give it a luxuriant healthy appearance and delay the inevitable loss due to age or heredity.

Medical treatments have recently become available. Applications of minoxidil (Rogaine) solution to the scalp twice a day results in improvement in about six months. Finasteride, is a pill which when swallowed regularly blocks the formation of the active male hormones in the hair follicle and causes hair growth in men. It cannot be used in women.

Hair transplantation is a time consuming expensive plastic surgery procedure. It is a permanent form of hair replacement, which can be used in men and women who have suffered permanent hair loss. It involves moving hair from donor sites on the head to recipient sites with simultaneous removal of the bald skin. The procedure is an expensive cosmetic alternative to augment scanty scalp hair.

For proper care and maintenance of normal hair a few tips need to be followed.

- ➢ Oil the hair twice a week using the tips of the fingers (not the nails).
- ➢ Massage the oil into the scalp.
- ➢ A homemade excellent combination consists of a mixture of
- ➢ ½ kilo coconut oil,
- ➢ ½ kilo sesame oil
- ➢ 100 ml castor oil

➤ Add a bunch of curry leaves, a clove and 20 peppercorns and boiled it in this mixture. If darkening of the hair is also required curry leaves, henna leaves or powder, and shoe flower petals (red hibiscus) can be boiled in the oil in addition.

➤ Wash the hair without chemicals. Use home made shikakai powder mixed with a soap nut (reeta) solution. All commercial shampoos and most packaged "ready to use" herbal powders have chemical and foaming additives which are likely to damage you hair. Packaged ready made shikakai powder also has chemical additives.

➤ Crinkling and curling can be safely done at home by plaiting the hair tightly and leaving it overnight. There is no need to use heat treatments and chemical curlers

➤ Blow-drying damages hair. If a dryer has to be used, cover the head with a towel and allow the air to heat the towel instead applying it directly to the head.

➤ Eat a nutritious diet with adequate protein (6 gm/day). Take regular supplements of vitamins, iron, zinc and calcium.

➤ Have split ends trimmed professionally.

With a little care your appearance will be striking.

Chapter 26

The Lowly Louse

The pamphlet stated that kerosene was the cheapest and most effective treatment for head lice; that it should be extensively applied to the whole scalp and left for 2–3 hours, after which it should be washed off with shampoo. That might be the case, but unless warned to stay away from fire, a tragic accident may result.

Head lice have co-existed with mankind all over the world, and they have frustrated all attempts at eradication for many centuries. Dead lice have even been found on Egyptian mummies.

Head lice are actually six-legged insects called Pediculus capitis. They have a brown waxy body and six long tapering legs with which they can move rapidly clinging to the hair shafts. They cannot fly or jump. They can efficiently crawl from one head to the next with sufficiently close contact. Specific types of lice infest different animals. Human lice cannot survive on dogs, cats and other pets. Neither can lice be transmitted by these animals. Even in the human, different types of lice infest different areas of the body. There are "body lice and "pubic lice" named after the specific area they inhabit. Lice from one area of the body cannot inhabit another.

Transmission from one human to another occurs only by close head contact, or by sharing helmets, towels, bed sheets and clothes. Head lice can also crawl along sheets, seats and furniture. They cannot survive for more than 24 hours without a meal of human blood. They can be killed by immersion in oil for two hours or more. They die if submerged in water for 6 hours. They can also be killed by boiling, hot air pesticides and chemicals.

Lice infesting the genital area (pubic lice) are sexually transmitted. They are known colloquially as "crab lice." They cannot survive on the head or on the rest of the body. Body lice are also different even though they belong to the same species. They spread during times of war and famine. They cause louse-borne typhus, louse-borne relapsing fever and trench fever.

Head lice cause itching and irritation. The constant scratching may disturb sleep and even keep the person awake. They may migrate to the eyelids and eye lashes. Their saliva and faeces may cause allergies and sensitize people to their bites. Scratching may cause secondary infection. The lymph nodes in the neck may become painful and enlarged mimicking infectious mononucleosis, tuberculosis or cancers. Head lice do not transmit infections from person-to-person. Lice are burdensome, a cause of annoyance and a social embarrassment, but they cannot really be considered a public health problem.

Lice infest the rich and poor alike. They do not reflect neglect on the part of the parents. They do not show class distinctions. Infestation is more common in school children and in the debilitated. Lice do not survive on people taking high doses of antibiotics. Antibiotic administration however is not a recommended treatment for the eradication of lice.

Lice multiply rapidly and within a few days cause an uncontrolled and embarrassing infestation. A cohabitating couple can produce 100 eggs in a lifetime. Each egg hatches after 8 days and develops into an adult stage in around 10 days.

Head lice infestation is diagnosed by inspection. The appearance may be confused with dandruff or seborrhic dermatitis.

In India we had certain traditional ways of tackling head lice without resorting to pesticides and chemicals.

➤ The whole family can be tonsured on the same day—no hair—no lice. This method removed the nits (eggs) as well.

➤ Take equal quantities of coconut oil and sesame oil. Place it is an iron kadai. Add neem and curry leaves, boil, cool and strain. Oil and then comb the hair, with a fine toothed comb. This makes the adult lice slip out.

➢ Nits can also removed by this method. The entire population may not be eradicated immediately, but if the procedure is repeated twice a week for several months the infestation is controlled.

Head lice can also be treated with chemicals called applied to the hair as creams, lotions or shampoos. Eggs usually survive chemical treatments. Reapplication of the chemical is required after 10 days to kill any newly hatched lice before they start to reproduce.

The head louse has survived for thousands of years. Only 17 % are now susceptible to the commonly used chemicals malathion, lindane and permethrin. The majority are resistant. These pediculicides fail to eradicate all lice, and they began to mutate, thrive and multiply in the presence of these chemicals. Higher concentrations offer no greater benefit. Instead they build up to toxic levels in children and in the environment. These chemicals are contraindicated for use in pregnant women and children below the age of one.

Instead of chemicals some people opt for herbal products. They may or may not work. Their composition and concentration are not regulated and their efficacy and safety is questionable.

Lice infestation is a family problem. Each family must formulate their own way of tackling this problem, with regular hair inspection, and combing the hair with a fine toothed comb after oiling.

Even in the USA and Britain "bug busting" combs are widely advertised, gaining in popularity as they are found to be safer than external applications of toxic chemicals.

Louse infestation is a hazard commonly encountered during school-days. It must be tackled methodically and regularly.

CHAPTER 27

BACK ACHE

Back Breaking Thoughts

We are animals and our human body is actually designed to walk on all fours like the rest of the animal kingdom. We were not supposed to stand upright and gaze at the stars.

Either due to evolution, or divine intervention, we contravened this efficient design and lifted ourselves up.

We have paid a price for an upright gravity defying lifestyle with 80% of human beings suffering from lumbago (lower back ache) at some time during the course of their life.

Our backs are made up of very small bones called the vertebrae piled one on top of the other sequentially. They are separated by discs containing water and gel and are supported on the sides by ligaments and muscles. In the upright position, the lower vertebrae bear the weight of the ones above and the additional effect of gravitational pull. Also in some of us a vestigial tail remains or the vertebrae of the lower back are imperfectly designed.

Since nerves to the legs and arms come out of the little spaces between the vertebrae; any pathological non-alignment therefore impinges on the nerves and causes pain.

Young children usually do not complain about aches and pains unless they see elders moaning and groaning and then begin to mimic them. School children begin to complain of backache and shoulder pain around the time they attend middle school. Very rarely is it due to an actual back pathology. A heavy school bag, asymmetrically balanced on one sagging shoulder, with an accompanying water bottle, skews the centre of gravity and causes muscle and ligament strain. School hours are long and involve prolonged seating. School furniture is often not ergo metrically designed. The bench may be of improper height and lacking proper back support. Feet may not quite reach the floor. Some schools make the children sit on the floor while alterations and repairs are going on. Homework is done sprawled on the floor or across a sofa, with no attention being paid to posture.

Women are at particular risk. Fashionable footwear (block heels, stilettos, platforms) shifts the centre of gravity, and balance requires abnormal positions and manoeuvres on the part of the spine. Pregnancy exaggerates the normal shallow "s" bend (lordosis) of the lumbar spine. Hormonal laxity allows the alignment to "slip" with a resultant backache that sometimes persists through life.

In people unused to physical labour, unconditioned muscles and ligaments cannot respond efficiently to the stress of lifting, resulting in backache.

Weight gain places additional stress on the spine, with each extra kilo resembling a permanently attached knapsack, to be carried during all waking hours.

As age advances, the water content of the intervertebral disc naturally decreases, causing shrinkage, fragility and decreased pliability. This in itself causes older people to "pull" their backs and injure themselves. Bones too become weaker as their calcium content decreases with increasing age. Older people become shorter as their vertebrae collapse on each other. All these conditions combine together and there is a predisposition to frequent backaches.

Investigations are usually not required initially during the first episode of backache. They should be undertaken if there are danger signals, such as a backache persisting for more than 6 months, weakness of leg muscles, paralysis, loss of bladder or bowel control, passage of bloody urine, headache and vomiting.

X-rays are usually normal in the initial stages. They reveal gross bony abnormalities which may take some time to develop. CT and MRI scans though expensive are more informative. They pick up early pathology. In addition some blood tests may be required to arrive at a diagnosis.

Most backaches resolve spontaneously in a few days. It therefore makes economic sense to "watch and wait," instead of proceeding with a plethora of expensive investigations.

Recovery is hastened with limited physical activity, painkillers, external support, sleeping on a firm surface and muscle relaxants.

Traction, intra articular injections and prolonged absolute bed rest have not been shown to help and may actually delay eventual recovery.

Attention should be paid to correctable reversible factors, like posture, footwear and furniture. With a little care and effort, many backaches can be prevented

The school bag should not be more than 10 % of the weight of the child. It should have padded straps and be placed over both shoulders and not fashionably slung over one shoulder. Any other weights like a water bottle (A litre of water weights a kilo) should be consciously alternated between the two shoulders. Seating and lighting arrangements at schools and at home should be reviewed and improved if required. Children under the age of 16 years should not be allowed to wear heels. Even older women should wear supportive well designed slippers and foot wear if their work involves prolonged standing or walking.

A conscious effort should be made to shed excess weight and maintain the BMI (body mass index wt in kg/ height in m2) below 25.

If work standing for prolonged periods, alternating the weight on the legs by placing them one at a time on a platform or stool is beneficial.

Footwear should be comfortable and practical. Heels should be avoided.

Handbags and briefcases should be alternated between the two shoulders.

Initially, alternating a task, like carrying groceries, sweeping or moping, between the two hands, may be clumsy and inefficient. Expertise and dexterity eventually develops and the benefits to the spine are tremendous. Heavy labour should definitely alternate between the two sides for the same reasons.

Pregnant woman should do pre and postnatal exercises to reduce back strain and rapidly regain the original shape and form of their spines.

Exercises to strengthen the spine are found in yoga, aerobics and in the martial arts. They can be learnt from books, instructors, television or by following instructions on a website.

With conscientious regular back exercises, for a few minutes a day, from the age of ten, reaching for the stars can be painlessly and pleasantly achieved with a ramrod straight back.

CHAPTER 28

ARTHRITIS—LIVING WITH ACHES AND PAINS

The over weight woman hauled her self up the stairs with her flabby arms using the banisters for support. "I ache all over, my joints are stiff, and, if it rains I can barely walk". Anxiously she continued, "It is not arthritis is it?"

The word arthritis means, "pain" and it is a generic term encompassing a wide spectrum of diseases. Around 60% of the population experiences a certain degree of pain at some time every year. Generally the incidence increases with age and it is commoner in women. By the age of 70, 90% of the populations of both sexes are affected.

All forms of arthritis cause pain swelling and disability. The sex and the predominant age group affected and the treatment are very different depending on the diagnosis of the arthritis.

Gout, caused by an inherited biochemical defect, is commoner in older males. Rheumatoid arthritis, on the other hand, is an autoimmune disease effecting mainly young women. The juvenile form of the same disease affects children. Ankylosing spondylitis (bamboo spine) is a hereditary disease seen in the young adult male. Fibromyalgia causes pain but joints are usually spared. The commonest form of arthritis is the degenerative joint disease called osteoarthritis.

The bones in the body are separated by joints and held in position by protective muscles and tendons. The ends of bones are prevented from rubbing against each other and producing grating friction by cartilage padding and lubrication with synovial fluid. As a result of wear and tear, the cartilage gets damaged. The ends of the bones are now in contact with each other producing a palpable crepitus, nerve ends are exposed producing excruciating pain, bits of bone break off forming "loose bodies, " and extra bone forms called "spurs."

All this results in inefficient functioning of the joints, incapacitating pain, interference with daily routine, misalignment, deformity and eventual immobility.

Damage automatically increases with years of usage and this in turn increases with age. X-rays and scans universally demonstrate osteoarthritic degenerative changes in bones after the age of 75 in 90% of the population. There are variations in the severity and expression of the disease. Many are spared pain and enjoy unrestricted physical activity despite having radiological osteoarthritis.

The extent of the disease is influenced by genetics, with earlier onset of osteoarthritis being transmitted in some families. It is commoner in women, in the obese (BMI over 25), the inactive, diabetics and smokers. It is also worsened by coexisting depression.

Arthritis is not confined to man alone, nor is it a twentieth century disease phenomenon. Evidence of osteoarthritis has been found in dinosaur fossils and mummified pharaohs. It has even ceased to be a disease of the senior citizens. It can occur in apparently fit young individuals, especially athletes, dancers and other professionals, whose jobs or lifestyle involve repetitive movements of a particular set of joints. There is an epidemic of CRI (Computer Related Injury) among young people employed in call centres, typists and data processors.

Timely medical advice and intervention can reduce and delay progression of the disease and ensuing joint deformity in all forms of arthritis.

> ➤ Reduce your weight so that the BMI remains below 25. (Your bones then no longer have to groan under the load they carry!)
>
> ➤ Inactivity increases disability. Walk or swim for 45 minutes a day.

- ➤ Do exercises to maintain muscle strength with a trained qualified physiotherapist. If this is not possible learn yoga or tai chi from classes, books or CDs. Strong muscles over a joint can be strengthened to hold it in place. This prevents misalignment by preventing bones from slipping and sliding.

- ➤ Medications can help, especially the NSAID group (Non Steroidal Anti Inflammatory Drugs). The older ones like aspirin, brufen piroxicam and naprosyn are relatively safe but have gastrointestinal side effects. The newer agents like diclofenac sodium damage the kidneys. Some COX-2 inhibitors occasionally cause fatal reactions and some can cause fatal cardiac arrhythmias in susceptible individuals.

- ➤ External applications of counter irritants like extracts of capsicum, liniments and herbal oils when combined with warm moist heat help relieve pain.

- ➤ Splints and external supports can be worn to prevent jarring and attendant pain. They are particularly useful while working or travelling.

Surgical interventions are popular but expensive. Intra-articular steroid in injections are effective. Repeated injections eventually destroy the joint. They should be given only by qualified individuals.

Arthroscopic surgery can be used to remove loose bodies and damaged cartilage.

Osteotomy realigns the deformed joint.

Arthodesis fuses the joint, preventing movement and hence pain.

Arthroplasty replaces an irretrievably damaged joint with an artificial joint.

The frantic pace of life in the 21 st century and the pursuit of gainful employment and academic laurels has resulted in a generation that does not exercise or remain sufficiently physically active to prevent arthritis from evolving and progressing. Monetary gain results in health loss.

Regular exercise can keep your body flexible pain free and fit, and provide enough stamina to complete the race in the marathon of life.

Chapter 29

Painful Heels

Wincing in anticipation from pain, the middle aged women placed her foot gingerly on the ground. The first step was absolute agony, sending sharp shooting pains all the way to her brain. It was like being struck by lightening.

This is a common scenario and it does not affect women exclusively. Many people, of all ages and both sexes suffer from pain in one or more heels.

Initially pain appears intermittently while running, jumping, or making quick turns. Eventually, it becomes constant and nagging and is worse after prolonged sitting or lying down. Even athletes experience similar discomfort. The only difference is that in them the pain is abrupt in onset and present continuously.

Heel pain is often due to an inflammation of a sturdy thick fibrous band of tissue called the plantar fascia, situated on the sole of the foot. This actually functions as an arch support and prevents flat feet. Pain occurs when this plantar fascia is stretched, usually as a result of overuse and overload. Small tears then occur in areas where the fascia meets the heel bone. If movements of the foot are also associated with tingling along sides of the foot then some of the nerves may also be entrapped under the thick fascia.

Pain in the heel may also arise as a result of stress and strain injuries in the Achilles tendon situated at the back of the heel. Over a lifetime, it contracts many million times while standing walking running and jumping.

Both types of heel pain tend to occur in people with congenital flat feet, or if they are obese or pregnant. Women sometimes are improperly balanced on footwear with high heels. Structural abnormalities of the foot can also be triggered by wearing shoes with poorly cushioned heels. The resulting abnormal gait causes the formation of an extra bony growth at the back of the heel. This soon leads to inflammation and pain.

Walking barefoot on hard and stony ground can cause trauma and injury to the back of the heel. A puncture wound can cause bacterial infection of the soft tissue around the heel which can spread to the bone. The infection can become serious if the blood supply to the foot is inadequate or if the person has poorly controlled diabetes.

Athletes, (runners, joggers volleyball and tennis players), and those who exercise using an aerobics or stair climbing program can develop painful heels. It may be due to intense training without proper stretching and warm up exercises. Improper footwear can also cause rupture of the tendon at the back of the ankle or a severe impact injury to the heel pad.

Active children between the ages of 8–14 who participate in sports involving jumping and running, can develop heel pain, especially if their sports shoes are ill-fitting or improper. This is because the repeated stress causes irritation of thegrowth centre in the middle of the heel.

Pain in the heel can occasionally be a manifestation of other diseases like diabetes, rheumatoid arthritis or gout.

X-rays may reveal a bony parrots beak like hooked growth at the base of the heel. This can provide an explanation for the heel pain. However, 10% of people without any pain have this growth. It is can be discovered incidentally during a routine x-ray.

To prevent pain in the heels:

➤ Maintain ideal body weight throughout life.

➤ Spare a few minutes to do stretching exercises morning and evening.

➤ Stand with the feet six inches apart. Raise your hands up over the head. With the knees straight and eyes fixed ahead reach for the stars.

➤ Stand on the right leg. Place the left foot on the back of the ankle. Raise the right foot and stand on the toes. Repeat on the other side.

➤ While exercising wear appropriate foot wear. Purchase sports shoes that are flexible and "give" easily, and are not rigid and stiff. If possible wear shoes with good padding or an air cushion in the heel.

➤ Once pain has occurred:

➤ Soak the foot in hot water with salt morning and evening for 10 mins.

➤ Then apply an ice pack to the heel for 10mins

➤ Stand on a cushion and rock back and forth a few times.

➤ Take a mild analgesic like ibubrufen or paracetemol.

➤ Take a single leaf of aloe vera, heat in on a tawa and apply to the affected heel.

If there is no improvement after a week of these simple home remedies then an expert orthopaedic evaluation is required.

Eventually, splints, supports, injections into the painful region or surgery may be required depending on the diagnosis.

To prevent the above unpleasant experiences and to stride forward confidently and painlessly, stretch and warm up every morning, irrespective of whether you are a young, school going , athletic, ill or elderly.

CHAPTER 30

CRI IN CHILDREN (COMPUTER RELATED INJURY)

The boy held his head held tilted to one side, stared blankly, and incessantly rubbed the thumb of his right hand. His tearing eyes blinked infrequently, his mouth was pursed and one shoulder drooped lower than the other.

What had reduced an active healthy eight-year old to this state?

His mother inadvertently provided the answer, "we bought him a computer. He has been working on it all day for the entire summer vacation."

Computers are the gateway to a better economic future for the individual, the family and country. With our multilingual society, knowledge of English, mathematical analytical brains and natural ability, we are poised to take over the cyber world. We now have an unprecedented access to personal computers (PCs) and children use them proficiently. They "learn computers "in school and "use" them at home. "Computer illiterate" parents provide "super fast" state of the art PCs for their children, loaded with "free" games and other soft ware. Using a computer seems to be more educative than passive viewing of the "cartoon network" and brain dead TV serials. Besides, the hazards of becoming an unhealthy television viewing "couch potato" been widely publicized.

Is it all that different?

These children lack physical activity. They are seated for long hours staring unblinkingly at a flickering computer screen. They are not making any earthshaking discovery. They are playing games, and in the process they develop hand eye coordination, anticipation, strategic planning, lateral thinking and quick reflexes.

The cost of this life style has only now begun to emerge.

Some children log on to the internet, join chat rooms, form "cyber-pals" with unknown IDs and log on to pornographic sites.

Children are seated at "computer workstations" manufactured and adjusted for adults. Their legs do not reach the floor, so the sitting position compromises blood supply to the legs. They are forced to strain their necks and shoulders as they stare awkwardly upwards at the monitor. With arms too short to reach the keyboard, they sit too close to the computer screen. The unfiltered glare causes eye fatigue and damage. Protective blinking is infrequent as the activity on the screen is too engrossing for even a split-second laxity. They drum at certain specific keys that operate the commands, or have their hands glued to a joystick or mouse. In hand held video games, the thumbs continuously perform unnatural hammer like movements. This may eventually cause "trigger fingers".

Adults can also suffer from computer related injuries (CRI) if proper workstation ergonomics are not followed. This fact has received wide publicity. Companies, facing lawsuits, have been legally compelled to deal with this problem. They provide medical evaluation, enforce regular breaks, teach relaxation techniques and purchase technically correct equipment.

Parents have to voluntarily recognize the unpublicized dangerous signals of childhood CRI, and then proceed to rectify the problem themselves. There is no legislation to enforce compliance.

> ➢ CRI is more dangerous in children than in adults as their growing malleable musculo-skeletal system is more susceptible to permanent and irreparable damage.

> ➢ Danger signals are heralded by the metamorphosis of a gregarious youngster into a uncommunicative child, with poor social skills, itchy tearing eyes, rubbing the backs of their hands and complaining of radiating pain in the shoulders or neck.

> ➤ Failure to promptly recognize these symptoms leads to progression with eventual deterioration in performing mundane tasks like writing, buttoning clothes or tying shoelaces.

Parents should try to search for suitable supervised physical activity for children during the summer vacation. Tennis camps, cricket coaching, swimming and athletic coaching is available in many towns and cities. Children should be encouraged to join these. Though they seem to be safe in the home environment, silently "working on the computer," parents should be aware that they are watching ticking time bombs.

It is not enough to take half-measures to prevent CRI as there is a complex interrelationship between the numerous risk factors. Addressing a few problems "because it's better than doing nothing" is not helpful, because a permanent, crippling injury could result from the guidelines that were ignored.

Prevention can be achieved by following a few principles:

> ➤ In schools, relevant facts should be brought to the notice of the authorities at parent teacher meetings.
>
> ➤ At home, children should not be given laptops for constant use.
>
> ➤ The monitor should face the child "head on" at eye level. It should not be skewed to one side..
>
> ➤ The glare of the screen should be reduced to a minimum.
>
> ➤ Computer tables and chairs should have adjustable heights. Children are smaller than adults. If there is more than one child then the furniture should be readjusted for each child.
>
> ➤ "Free" movements of the wrist and fingers should be used, instead of being rested on angulated support pads.
>
> ➤ The posture should be closely monitored.
>
> ➤ Every twenty minutes of computer activity should be followed by an "active" five-minute break with standing, stretching and wrist and arm movements.

There should be a minimum of 30 minutes of daily aerobic activity preferably jogging outdoors. Interaction with peers and friendships should be encouraged as "computer geeks" moult into socially inept adults, unable to adjust and function in society or the workplace.

The factors causing injury are interrelated, complex, physical and psychological. Half measures and compromises will not help. It could be your child that develops permanent crippling "work related injury" to their physique and psyche even before entering the work force, because of inadvertently ignored risk factors!

Chapter 31

Cancer—The Frightening Big C

"If you have no time for exercise, you better reserve a lot of time for disease."

No one suddenly gets cancer, yet everyone is afraid of the word. Sometimes it seems as though there is an epidemic, as everyone knows some one who has been diagnosed to have cancer. With the increasing global population, even if the percentage diagnosed with cancer increase marginally, it has a tremendous impact on the total numbers.

Actually, cancer has been around for centuries. Now, it seems to be more prevalent, as physicians are more aware of the disease and its manifestations. All kinds of blood tissue and imaging tests are available. Diagnostic procedures are quick accurate. The disease is picked up in early stages, sometimes at the microscopic cellular level.

In our journey through life on the planet, our bodies are exposed externally and internally to a variety of natural and artificial substances. Some of these cause biochemical and microscopic changes at the cellular level. These may become cancerous at a later stage. Often, several years pass before symptoms develop after exposure to the noxious stimulus. There are many types of cancer which may affect various different organs and tissues of the body. Cancers also may take a long time to develop to the visible size or the symptomatic stage.

Each person's body responds differently to a harmful stimulus. This makes establishing a cause and effect relationship in cancer more difficult than is the case in other diseases, where the end result is immediately seen.

The cells in our body are being constantly replenished. Sometimes, uncontrolled multiplication of a few cells produces an overgrowth of tissue. It can develop into a harmless or benign growth with microscopically normal tissue, or a cancerous tumour with immature and bizarre cells.

Common risk factors for the development of cancer are the use of tobacco products, carcinogens (toxic chemicals) in the work environment, lack of exercise, an improper diet and a family history of cancer. Genes cannot be changed. Awareness of a familial or genetic susceptibility to a certain kind of cancer should lead to an attempt to minimize other aggravating factors.

The influence of diet on disease has been known for centuries. The old saying, "an apple a day keeps the doctor away, "has a scientific basis. Fruits and vegetables contain cancer fighting and blocking phytochemicals, called phenols, indols, flavones, cumines, and isothiocyanates. Phytoestrogens from plant foods, like cauliflower and cabbage, block oestrogen receptor sites on cells and lower the risk of oestrogen-dependent cancers, such as breast cancer.

Eating raw fruits and vegetables is filling, suppressing the appetite and the desire to consume high calorie, oil and animal fat saturated snacks. Such snacks increase the risk of cancer. The high fibre content in raw natural food also prevents constipation and decreases contact between some carcinogenic food particles and intestinal cells, protecting them. A diet containing yellow and red fruits and vegetables is also rich in antioxidants, beta carotene, vitamin C and vitamin E. These protect the membrane of intestinal cells, neutralize carcinogenic free-radical reactions and prevent faulty metabolism in the cell itself, reducing the risk of cancer. Good sources of beta carotene are carrots, melons, pumpkins, spinach, mango, and papaya.

Soya contains the chemical isoflavone which inhibits the growth of new blood vessels necessary for tumour survival. However, soya also contains phyto estrogens and so should be taken in moderation, a tablespoon or so a few times a week. It is available as flakes, chunks, milk and sauce. They must however be avoided by patients with sex hormone dependent tumours or a family history of such disorders.

For non vegetarians, sea food is rich in protective omega 3 fatty acids. Chicken is safer than red meat like mutton, pork or beef. A high incidence of colon and prostate cancer is found in populations that eat red meat. Cooking meat by grilling it produces some well done and burnt portions. Grilling can release carcinogenic cellular DNA damaging chemicals into the meat. Poaching, stewing, baking and slow low-heat cooking is safer and releases fewer carcinogens. Consumption of microwaved food does not increase the risk of cancer.

Calcium controls the uncontrolled multiplication of epithelial cells lining the colon, binds cancer-producing bile acids, keeps them from irritating the colon, and decreases the risk of cancer. An average intake of 1,200 mg. of calcium a day is recommended. Good sources of calcium are dairy products, like milk and curds and bony fish.

While cooking, reduce oil consumption to 1 tsp of oil per person per day as far as possible. Use monounsaturated oils, or a mixture of oils. This is safer than saturated and hydrogenated oils and fats.

Garlic and turmeric used in traditional cooking have been found to have some cell protective properties.

Alcohol, especially beer contains pre-carcinogenic nitrosamines, which can be activated in the intestines and has been linked to colon cancer. Red wine contains harmful tannins.

Exercise improves metabolic efficiency. Muscle mass activated during exercise burns fat and lowers cholesterol. Exercise also increases the production and efficiency of disease fighting chemicals called interleukins, and of certain kinds of white blood cells called lymphocytes and "killer" T cells. These destroy cancer cells. Exercise increases the efficiency of the intestines, so that transit time for food products is reduced and ingested carcinogens are rapidly cleared from the body.

Active people, who use more than 2500 calories a week with exercise, have a 50% less chance of developing cancer when compared to their couch potato peers. The lowest rates of cancer are found in fit people with a slow resting heart rate. Even if cancer occurs, a physically fit individual is able to withstand and survive the surgery, radiation and curative medication required for treatment.

Expending 2500 calories a week for a 60 kg adult requires walking or cycling for an hour, running or continuous swimming for 45 minutes, or stair climbing for 20 minutes, at least 6 days a week.

Cancer risk can be reduced by::

- ➤ Exercise sufficiently to overcome the body's battle against renegade cancer cells:
- ➤ Prayer and meditation to reduce stress.
- ➤ Maintenance of ideal body weight.
- ➤ Limit dietary fat and eliminate hydrogenated fats.
- ➤ Increase dietary fibre.
- ➤ Eat fruits and vegetables
- ➤ Avoid red meat
- ➤ Eat seafood and soy products.
- ➤ Eat foods high in calcium.

A diagnosis of cancer is no longer a death sentence. Cancer is not necessarily fatal, and now there are efficient curative and palliative medical surgical and radiation treatments.

Once the diagnosis is made, seek treatment in a reputed specialized cancer centre as soon as possible. It is better to avoid unscientific unsubstantiated anecdotal treatment from unqualified quacks.

With courage, motivation and finances you can treat and outlive your cancer.

CHAPTER 32

STERILITY, PRIMARY OR SECONDARY

"Childless, desperate, living in hell."

"I am not pregnant!" The face is woebegone, the stance droopy the demeanour depressed. "I have been married for four months now."

Why are couples so desperate when it comes to reproduction?

Is it a desire to transmit genes to a future generation?

Or is it the reason more mundane? Being sidelined at birthday parties, school functions, and ignored by child rearing friends? Being considered an unwelcome presence at auspicious occasions like marriages and engagements?

In India, marriages are often a mutual contract between two strangers arranged by relatives with the help of matrimonial advertisements, marriage brokers and recently the internet. An unwritten but essential part of the negotiation is rapid procreation. Failure to fulfil this part of the obligation is a serious subtly punishable offence! The bride's family feels inadequate and guilty and the girl's family betrayed. Suspicions are aroused—Is the girl not normal? Were they hiding something? Or, even worse, is she secretly using contraception or inducing abortions?

These suspicions become paranoia if the woman has irregular periods, or is on regular medication for an unexplained or undisclosed chronic ailment. There is something suspect about a woman who secretly swallows undisclosed tablets every day or menstruates irregularly after delayed periods.

Around 10% of the Indian women in the child-bearing age have PCOS (polycystic ovarian Syndrome). Many of them have irregular periods and require tablets to menstruate. This arouses even greater suspicion, as a period of amenorrhoea is followed by tablet ingestion and menstruation.

Unfortunately many do have this problem of irregular periods from their late teens. Families anxious that no word should leak out, either blithely believes that "everything will be all right after marriage", or takes unregulated alternative medications. No attempt is made at analysing the problem or reaching a diagnosis.

Clinically, once these girls get married, infertility is a "failure to conceive" (become pregnant) after a year of unprotected sex (without the use of contraceptives).

In most couples in another year without any intervention or tests spontaneous pregnancy will occur. Patience and watchful anticipation are all that is needed!

Two people are involved in producing a baby. Statistics show that in cases of infertility, 40% of the time the male needs treatment, 40 % of the time it is the female partner and in 20%, both need medical management. Treatment of the woman alone is therefore likely to fail as she may actually be the normal partner.

Women release ova (eggs) from one of two ovaries once month, around the 14th day of the cycle. The egg drops into the fallopian tube, where it is ready for fertilization. Once the sperm enters the fallopian tube, it can survive for up to three days. Fertilization of the egg can occur at any point during that time. An unfertilized egg only survives 12 to 24 hours. Once fertilized, the egg moves into the uterus two to four days later where it is implanted and begins its nine-month growth into a baby. If pregnancy does not occur menstruation occurs 14 days after the release of the egg.

The highest rate of natural conception occurs if intercourse scheduled around the day of ovulation. If intercourse does not occur on those days, due to travel or work, years can pass without conception. This occurs when husband lives elsewhere, intercourse occurs infrequently (once a week or 2–3 times a month) and the woman's fertile period is missed. Conception fails to occur even though both partners on examination are physically and physiologically normal.

Women do not to function like machines. A normal woman can have menstrual cycles which vary in length, making mathematical calculations for fertile dates imprecise. Ovulation occurs 14 days before the next period, NOT 14 after the previous period. This fine distinction becomes important if the cycles are 30-35-37- 45 days and not a regular lunar calendar schedule of 28 days. Unless intercourse is regular and frequent, it is possible the fertile days can be missed entirely for years.

Once a couple has decided on medical advice and fertility intervention, the preliminary screening involves a physical examination of both partners and a semen analysis for the male. At this stage certain correctable factors can be tackled.

A BMI (wt in kg / height in meters square) greater than 25 or less than 14 needs correction, as the metabolism of the hormones required for fertility are affected by the fat content of the body. Both gross under nutrition or over nutrition can cause a reproductive "shut down."

- ➤ Food faddists may have difficulties conceiving if they lack important nutrients in their diet, such as vitamin B12, zinc, iron, and folic acid. Alcohol intake (as little as 150 ml a week), and caffeine found coffee, tea, colas, chocolate, can cause relative infertility if consumed in excess.

- ➤ Male smokers have lower sex drives, lower sperm counts and poorer sperm quality than non-smokers. Their sperms often do not move fast or are abnormal.

- ➤ Prior radiation or chemotherapy for cancer in either partner reduces fertility.

- ➤ Certain sexual practices, like incomplete penetration, coitus interruptus (ejaculation of the sperm outside the vagina) and douching after intercourse decreases the risk of pregnancy. The patient may be ignorant and unaware of correct sexual techniques.

- ➤ Relative infertility occurs in persons (men and women) employed in the tobacco industry or if they are exposed to high doses of pesticides and other chemicals.

> ➢ Treatable diseases adversely a affecting fertility in the female are sexually transmitted diseases, pelvic tuberculosis, pelvic inflammatory disease, chronic appendicitis, ruptured appendix, septic abortions, endometriosis and the polycystic ovarian syndrome (PCOS).

> ➢ Sometimes any of the above conditions can cause a block in the fallopian tubes preventing the fertilized egg from reaching the uterus.

These causes are easily diagnosed, correctable and treatable.

Despite simple interventions, 20% of the couples remain infertile a year later. At this point specialized treatment is needed.

Fertility interventions are based on science and fact and not on native medicines, magical potions, folk lore, luck and other quackery. There are many centres offering fertility interventions, but before embarking on treatment some preliminary investigations should be done. Unscientific hit or miss therapy is not advisable.

The success rate of the chosen centre should be evaluated and the qualifications of the doctors checked. Remember promotional gimmicks and public advertisements in newspapers, buses and trains are unethical. They should be viewed with suspicion.

The authenticity, integrity, honesty and ethical practices of the centre should be investigated before a decision is made. Frequent consultations and hospital visits may be required, so the distance to be travelled, finance and confidence in the medical personnel involved should be considered. If finances are not a constraint, and a baby "at any cost" the only driving factor, several centres offer artificial insemination (donor or husband), and test tube babies.

Any intervention undertaken should, be with complete knowledge, written consent, adequate documentation and confidentiality. If these criteria are not fulfilled it is better to go elsewhere to safeguard the health of both the mother and that of the unborn child.

Reproducing couples are not functioning in a time constrained factory production line! They should want to have a baby and not proceed half heartedly for treatment because of pressure from relatives an dwell-wishers.

Reproduction is a normal physiological process which takes longer in some couples even when they try obeying the adage "go forth and multiply."

Chapter 33

Polycystic Ovarian Syndrome

"She has really changed"

Sometimes a beautiful svelte girl changes during her teenage years. She unexpectedly becomes fat, especially around the waist, and develops an unsightly paunch. Her smooth skin becomes oily, and spotted with disfiguring acne. Hair appears on the face, neck, arms, hands, breasts, or thighs. The hair on the scalp becomes scanty with male pattern baldness. Patches of thickened dark brown or black skin may appear on the neck, arms, armpits and thighs. This makes her look like she has been negligent about her hygiene and has not bothered to take a proper bath. Tiny excess flaps of skin (skin tags) appear in the armpits or neck hanging like extra digits. Sometimes these get snarled in clothing causing pain and discomfort.

She often becomes self conscious, aware that her figure and looks do not fit in with the concept of the Indian beauty, tall, fair, thin, shapely doe eyed and clear complexioned . Her unsightly paunch makes form-fitting clothing a distant dream. Her family starts to get irritated as her loud snoring disturbs everyone's sleep.

These girls may complain of irregular, scanty or absent menstruation. Sometimes there is no bleeding for months; only to be followed by heavy bleeding that does not stop. There may be pain in the lower abdomen, which may be continuous or intermittent. Even touching the abdomen may be painful. Sometimes the pain occurs during the periods (dysmenorrhoea) and may be incapacitating.

In India 5–10% of the women in the child bearing (14–40) have varying degrees of this problem. They suffer from the polycystic ovarian syndrome (PCOS). This used to be called PCOD (polycystic ovarian disease) or the Stein Leventhal syndrome, until modern investigative techniques made physicians realize that the polycystic ovaries were only part of a wider spectrum of biochemical abnormalities, similar to "syndrome X."

Recognition of the physical changes is important for early intervention. The diagnosis is based on a high degree of suspicion. Usually other women in the family may be affected, or, one or both parents may be diabetic. There is no absolute diagnostic test for PCOS. There may be high blood sugars, high cholesterol, high blood pressure and higher level of male hormones. These are not essential for the diagnosis. An ultrasound scan of the abdomen usually clinches the diagnosis revealing multiple fluid filled cysts in both ovaries.

Women have two ovaries, one on each side of the single uterus. The ovaries have tiny sacs called follicles that hold eggs. Although each month about 20 eggs start to mature, only one becomes dominant, grows, accumulates fluid and eventually breaks open. This process, called ovulation, releases the egg for fertilization.

In women with PCOS, the ovarian hormones are inadequate and the eggs fail to mature fully. In addition the covering (skin) of the ovary tends to become abnormally thick. No one egg becomes large enough. Instead, they remain as fluid filled cysts. Ovulation does not occur and the menstrual cycle becomes irregular, prolonged or absent. Eggs have to produced and released for babies. In the absence of ovulation, fertility is affected, and these women do not become pregnant.

The insulin produced by these women is ineffective and may be defective. They also have a relatively high insulin resistance. Food eaten is not metabolized properly and is converted into fat deposited around the midriff causing the appearance of an unsightly paunch. The ovaries respond to this relative hyperinsulinaemia with a disproportionate production of male hormones. Most of the physical changes of the syndrome can be explained by the alteration of the normal ratio between male and female hormones in women.

Concerned by the menstrual irregularities, unaware of the reasons, and worried by the social stigma, parents shop for a cure. Emboldened by the fact that other women in the family have similar problems with no obvious detrimental health effects, treatment is delayed. No investigations are done, and these girls are often randomly put on iron supplements or calcium tablets. They are told that both they and their reproductive organs are "weak". High calorie "strengthening" food is given, making the problem worse. Sometimes herbs, native medicines or Siddha tonics are taken. These may be prescribed by allopathic practitioners who have no clear idea about their actions or side effects. Some of these non-allopathic medications and "gynaecological tonics" are aggressively promoted by the pharma industry. Doctors are verbally assured that they will work for all "women's problems." This shot gun therapy may do more harm than good.

Treatment for PCOS is symptomatic, not curative. It is required to decrease the facial hair, reduce the weight, regularize the menstrual cycles and restore fertility. Before embarking on any treatment, it is essential that the diagnosis be confirmed by an ultrasound scan of the abdomen.

> ➢ Birth control pills (oral contraceptive pills) can regulate menstrual cycles, reduce male hormone levels, and help to clear acne. Women on the "OC pill" do not become pregnant. If the pill is stopped, the cycles become abnormal again. Some girls are unwilling to swallow OCPs as they fear the social stigma of being labelled promiscuous.

> ➢ A progesterone only pill can regulate the menstrual cycle. It does not help reduce acne and hair growth. It can be given continuously or for the last 7-10-14 days of the cycle.

> ➢ Metformin, is actually an anti-diabetic medication. It helps with PCOS symptoms. It not only corrects the relative insulin resistance, it also decreases the male hormone production, decreasing abnormal hair growth. It helps regulate and reduce the weight. Ovulation may spontaneously return after a few months. The use of metformin does not precipitate diabetes. Nor does a normal person on metformin develop hypoglycaemia.

➢ Women with PCOS require fertility medications to induce ovulation. The woman obviously has a problem with ovulation and the eggs are not being released. This does not necessarily mean that she is married to a normal partner. Before administering pills (clomiphene) and injections (gonadotropins) to stimulate ovulation, the husband's sperm count should be checked. Many couple erroneously work on the assumption that if one partner is abnormal the other need not be evaluated.

➢ During fertility treatment metformin should be continued as by tackling the insulin resistance it helps to reduce the dosage of fertility medication.

➢ A woman who is not planning to get pregnant can use spironolactone or combination of cyproterone acetate with hormonal pills to reduce hair growth on the body.

➢ Surgery (ovarian drilling) can be done to induce ovulation. It used to be a popular method of tackling the problem before the availability of ovulation inducing medication.

PCOS predisposes to other problems as well. The hormonal imbalance increases the risk of eventually developing endometrial (uterine lining) hyperplasia or cancer. The metabolic abnormalities contribute to the risk of developing diabetes, high cholesterol, high blood pressure, and heart disease.

Women with PCOS do become pregnant with treatment. The fertility interventions predispose them to multiple births (twins, triplets) and they may deliver prematurely. They have a higher incidence of abortions. They tend to develop complications like diabetes or hypertension during pregnancy. Metformin reduces these complications in pregnancy and also limits weight gain.

As women with PCOS reach menopause, the menstrual cycle may become more normal. However, excessive hair growth continues, and male pattern baldness or thinning hair may become worse after menopause.

With a little determination and effort these metabolic abnormalities can be corrected without medication. If weight is maintained in the normal range with diet and exercise, many of the hormonal abnormalities correct themselves. A reduction of as little as 10 % of the body weight can make the menstrual cycles more regular in women with PCOS. Women with PCOS have to eat less and exercise more than their normal counterparts.

Refusing second helpings, climbing stairs, walking and 40 minutes of aerobic activity daily in our female teenagers can go a long towards controlling the symptoms, manifestations, and misery of this common condition before it spirals out of control.

Chapter 34

Pregnancy Testing and Confirming Pregnancy

With 1.2 billion Indians and still counting— one would assume that Indians are experts in this sphere, but unfortunately this is not the case.

A frequent query is, "If a woman's periods do not appear on time is she pregnant"?

It is a strong possibility, if the woman is sexually active, not using reliable contraception and in the fertile age group (10–50 years.)

Periods do not necessarily have to be delayed or missed to diagnose pregnancy. Breast feeding women may not menstruate and yet may become pregnant. The converse can also occur and confound; a woman may continue to menstruate for a couple of months even after she is pregnant!

"I only had sex once! How can I be pregnant?"

This oft repeated statement has a ring of truth. Pregnancy can occur with a single act of sex, even if penetration has been incomplete, especially if the act took place in the fertile period. This is the few days around the release of the egg or ovulation. It is calculated as 14 days before the next period, and NOT as 14 days after the first day of the last period. This difference is subtle, but it can make a lot of difference if the person regularly has a longer 35 – 45 or 60 day cycle.

A delayed period may be viewed with trepidation or joy depending on the social circumstances of the woman. The reaction varies, depending on whether the woman has been anxiously trying to conceive, or is a single woman who has made a mistake, or a married woman with a complete family who became careless about contraception.

Irrespective, the period of watchful anticipation and anxiety has now been cut short with the advent of the new, easy, reliable and quick home pregnancy tests. A trip to the laboratory, hand carrying a drippy bottle of urine, or an embarrassing visit to a strange toilet to collect a sample, or a confessional visit to a doctor is no longer required.

The commercially available home pregnancy tests vary in cost from Rs 20 to Rs 60. The can be purchased in any medial shop over the counter (OTC). A few precautions however should be followed.

> While doing a test, the strip has to be brought to room temperature.

> It should be placed on a flat surface.

> The instructions carefully followed. Usually, it involves collection a sample of urine in a clean bottle, then drawing up urine with the dropper provided, and placing the required number of drops (usually 3), in the demarcated area on the strip.

> After the specified reaction time (usually 5 minutes) the result appears. It is usually 2 lines, a test and a control, either pink or blue in colour. The result is easy to read, with two lines (however faint) indicating a positive result and one line a negative one. If the test is scrutinized after a longer period, evaporation of the urine may produce a confusing appearance.

The line that appears shows a reaction to the hormone HCG (Human Chorionic Gonadotropin) produced by the implanted embryo. The secretion of this hormone is highest in the morning and that is probably the best time to do the test. At other times, excessive fluid consumption may make the urine is too dilute and give a false negative result.

The test is positive only after implantation of the fertilized ovum. It is positive on the first day after the missed period in 90 % of the women, and in 97% after a week. Since ovulation occurs approximately 14 days before the period, by the time the pregnancy is confirmed, the ovum is 14 or more days old.

If for any reason the pregnancy is unplanned, unwanted or a mistake, do not wait longer in the vain hope that somehow menstruation will spontaneously occur. Confirm the result and know your status so that decisions can be made.

Sometimes the results of the tests may be equivocal. There may be faint lines, or the control line "c" may not appear. In this case read the instructions again to see if you performed the test correctly.

If it is still doubtful, wait for 2 days and check again. Alternatively, you can proceed to do a blood test for Beta HCG levels. This is available in most laboratories, and is relatively expensive, but it is more accurate, as it measures the HCG levels in the blood.

After the 1 st trimester (14 weeks after the last menstrual period) the HCG levels start to drop. In later pregnancy the test may not be reliable.

A false positive does not occur with oral contraceptive pills, progesterone tablets or injections or clomiphene tablets. False positive (chemical pregnancy) results can occur if the test is done within 8 weeks of a delivery or abortion. It can also occur if HCG injections have been given as a part of infertility treatment or for some other medical indication. The medicine should be stopped for 7–10 days and the test repeated. Alternatively a scan should be done to confirm the presence or absence of a pregnancy. This will prevent stress, tension and false hopes.

A delayed period during the reproductive years should be taken seriously irrespective of the situation. Women are sometimes caught unawares, or may suffer contraceptive failure. A dose of oral contraceptive may have been forgotten. (Always count the pills taken and check the pack). An IUCD (Intrauterine contraceptive device) can fail even though it is 99.2–99.9% effective. A condom though 60 % effective when used may leak or burst. Males practising withdrawal may have loose control and ejaculate earlier than anticipated. The safe period (the part of the menstrual cycle when pregnancy is least likely to occur) may have been wrongly calculated. Pregnancy can rarely (less than 0.01%) occur after surgical sterilization of either partner with tubectomy or vasectomy.

Sometimes "spotting" of blood may occur around the time the period is due, misleading the woman. This is due to the ovum burrowing into the uterine lining during implantation. It is not a "light" period. If in doubt, then it is better to repeat the test after 4–5 days. Sometimes spotting may be due to the implantation of the foetus taking place in an abnormal region like the tubes. This can cause severe pain and is dangerous if it bursts. If there is pain, a physician should be contacted immediately.

Accompanying symptoms of early pregnancy reinforce the diagnosis, but are not fool proof. Although nausea and vomiting have long been touted as the classical symptoms of pregnancy, actually the commonest are lassitude, drowsiness and unexplained fatigue. A previously active and energetic woman is tired sleepy, unfocussed and lethargic. Sometimes these symptoms set in before the period is missed or pregnancy suspected. This can confound the attending physician and lead to investigations for jaundice, and other causes for vomiting and malaise.

Classically vomiting due to pregnancy occurs in the morning, and is called "morning sickness", but this is not a hard and fast rule. It can occur at any time during the day. In most women vomiting stops by the 3rd month. In some others it continues till the bitter end, and after vomiting a last time, they deliver the baby!

Some of the conditions peculiar to pregnancy increase the vomiting, causing dehydration and making the patient sick enough to require admission. This hyperemesis may be due to infections, especially in the urinary tract or a gastritis. It can be precipitated by multiple foetuses (twins, triplets), or hydramnios, (excess amount of water in the uterus), or if the pregnancy itself does not develop normally, or forms a mass of tissue called a "mole" instead.

Pica (perverted appetite for non food items) is accepted internationally as "normal" during pregnancy. Pregnant women have been known to eat paint, chalk, powdered glass, dirt and chalk. Pica can he harmful. It is not peculiar to pregnancy, but it may be aggravated by it. It is usually a manifestation of nutritional deficiency of iron, zinc or calcium and responds rapidly to treatment. Unfortunately vomiting sometimes interferes with the treatment as the pregnant woman is unable to swallow the prescribed nutritional supplements.

Although the cause of these strange symptoms have not been biochemically explained, small frequent meals and snacking on salted carbohydrates helps.

Some women confound everyone by having no symptoms at all. This does not refute the diagnosis of pregnancy. They are just lucky!

Although pregnancy is a normal physiological process care has to be taken for its smooth progression and a healthy outcome.

Weight gain during pregnancy and an enlarging belly tends to cause unsightly stretch marks over thighs, breasts and abdomen. Many commercial preparations are available to over come this problem. A home made mixture of

500 ml of coconut oil,

500 ml of sesame oil and

100 ml of olive oil should be applied half an hour before bathing regularly from the beginning of pregnancy to prevent this before it occurs. At the same time the nipples should be gently pulled out using the same oil to prevent cracks and retraction during lactation.

Women deciding to get pregnant should finish their immunizations for MMR (measles mumps rubella) and hepatitis B before embarking on the adventure. Parents should try to make sure that these immunizations are complete before "arranging a marriage." Failure to give these immunizations means that the woman may acquire these diseases during pregnancy. German measles (rubella) and mumps are particularly dangerous in early pregnancy. They can cause abortion, miscarriage, intrauterine death or the birth of children with defects like blindness, deafness, congenital heart disease, mental retardation.

Cats should not be kept as pets during pregnancy.. They carry and transmit the infection toxoplasmosis which can cause serious abnormalities in the foetus.

Folic acid should be taken as early as possible; preferably from the time the decision to become pregnant is taken, as it prevents neural tube defects. Children of women deficient in folic acid can have abnormalities ranging from anencephaly (no skull) to spina bifida, (the failure of fusion in the midline of the spinal vertebrae). Part of the brain or spinal cord may protrude outside. There may be paralysis or weakness particularly of the lower limbs and urinary bladder.

If a regular exercise program was followed prior to pregnancy, it can be maintained during pregnancy with an appropriate reduction in the intensity. A woman unaccustomed to exercise should start very slowly and be careful about overexertion. Proper footwear should be worn, exhaustion avoided, hydration maintained and injuries prevented. Avoid exercises which involve lying flat on the back.

Women who exercise during pregnancy have better health, reduced weight gain; fewer mood swings and better sleep. Strong muscles and a fit heart can greatly ease labour and delivery. Gaining control over breathing helps manage and tolerate pain. If labour is prolonged, increased endurance is an advantage. On an average, in a woman who exercises regularly, labour is faster; with less need for anaesthesia or surgical intervention. Weight gained during pregnancy is also shed faster. Regular exercise promotes health and well-being in pregnancy. It does not increase the risk for miscarriage.

Pregnancy is not a disease, so eat a healthy well balanced diet make staying fit a priority.

Enjoy your pregnancy. Hopefully you will not go through it more than twice!

CHAPTER 35

EXERCISE IN PREGNANCY

Women, the more durable model made from a rib.

"Remember as a woman you have all the knowledge and power you need to give birth and to nurture your baby. It is in your genes. it has been there since you yourself were conceived."

God first made man, and something was missing. The reproductive function was just not complete. He realized that a physiologically stronger, more versatile and durable model was needed and made woman. He protected her by giving her double XX genes, in her chromosomes. This ensured that a weakness inherited from one parent was compensated by the normal complementary gene from the other.

Traditionally, men foraged for food, resting between hunting and farming. Women on the other hand really had no "time off". They helped with the male tasks, kept house and collected water, and in addition produced many children at short intervals. They were all active till the end of pregnancy.

All this activity made women healthy, with strong thigh and back muscles. They developed endurance, stamina and the determination to survive and rear their children in a hostile world. These physically fit and strong women delivered children normally. The weak and unfit women did not live to become adults. Sometimes, with no high tech medical interventions available, they died of complications during labour.

Times and traditional roles have changed. Women now lead sedentary lives. Fitness for girls is not a priority either in their youth or in later life. Only a lucky few are able to exercise.

Walking or jogging on the road requires grit, determination and a thick skin to ignore sexual innuendoes and sneering remarks from male passers by. Girls are admonished not to "go out" by family members, and to stay within the confines of the house or on the terrace, walking in boring vertigo inducing circles.

Although gyms are available on practically every street corner, they are expensive, and often the exclusive timings reserved for women are inconvenient. The family may refuse permission to join.

Women who wish to exercise are denied proper attire by well-meaning families, further reducing their motivation to remain fit. They find it difficult to exercise in cumbersome all-enveloping garments. They are not provided proper foot wear and are encouraged to "walk in their slippers."

These physically unfit women then become pregnant. This natural state is viewed as a terminal debilitating illness. There is a constant barrage of well-meaning but medically unsound advice to "take rest and lie down". Constant rest and lack of exposure to fresh air increases vomiting, backache, depression, and illnesses associated with pregnancy.

Eventually, an already flabby, unfit (though not necessarily fat) woman then embarks on the greatest adventure of her life, with no preparation, mental strength, physical stamina, endurance, or muscle tone to help her through the process.

Conception, delivery and motherhood will be easier if exercise and active participation in group and competitive sports for girls is started at the primary school level and then continued until formal education is completed (around the age of 22). Walking/jogging should be encouraged on a daily basis after that . Girls should try to achieve and maintain a BMI (Body Mass Index: weight divided by the height in meter squared) between 25 and 27 all through life.

Pregnant women should exercise regularly. Walking at a steady pace for 45 minutes both morning and evening is safe and beneficial. The road just in front of the house is a safe well-traversed territory. Just walk up and down. A treadmill is a good indoor alternative. If confined to a house or flat, mark a figure of 8 with a piece of chalk on the floor. Walk along the lines, clock wise and then anti-clockwise. The other alternative is to spot walking or marching while watching television or listening to music. All these though satisfactory are not a patch on "the real thing". They are better than no exercise at all.

Competitive sports like basket ball, tennis and badminton should be avoided when pregnant as there is a chance of falling and injuring the baby.

One of the fears frequently expressed about exercise during pregnancy is that it will in some way induce an abortion. Actually, a normal pregnancy with a healthy foetus will not be aborted by exercise. If a foetus is unhealthy, not growing normally or has abnormal genes, it is unlikely that it will proceed to term irrespective of whether the woman exercises or not! (There are actually only a few conditions during pregnancy when rest is advised by the obstetrician).

In addition to walking, muscle strengthening exercises should be performed.

➤ Kegel's exercises strengthen the perineum, which is most likely to tear during labour. These are done by consciously contracting the muscles needed to stop urine flow in mid-stream, for a count of four. Ten sets should be done at a time, three times a day.

➤ Pelvic tilt (angry cat). Get down on your hands and knees, arms shoulder-width apart and knees hip-width apart, keeping your arms straight. Tighten the abdominal muscles and tuck the buttocks under and around your back, breathing in. Relax and breathe out.

➤ Squat using a chair for support. Hold the squatting position for account of 10. Repeat 3 times.

➤ Sit cross-legged with your back against a wall for as long as possible.

➤ Warrior 2 pose: Stand with your feet apart. Raise your arms parallel to the floor and reach them actively out to the sides, palms down. Turn your right foot in slightly to the right and your left foot out to the left.. Stretch the arms parallel to the floor.

➢ Thai goddess pose: Sit on the floor with your buttocks resting on your heels and your left toe over your right. Hold for a count of 30.

➢ Cobbler pose: Sit up straight against a wall with the soles of your feet touching each other. Gently press your knees down and away from each other (do not force them apart) and stretch as long it is comfortable.

➢ The Lamaze exercises are excellent and can be learnt at home using a visual DVD or CD available at book and music stores.

Some of the higher-end gyms offer professional "birthing classes". The fees are high, and benefit has to be weighed against cost.

Exercising during pregnancy mainly requires information, motivation and a great deal of enthusiasm.

Listen to your body. Do not exercise to the point of pain. Do not do anything you find uncomfortable.

Exercising in pregnancy has several benefits. The weight gain is less, they have shorter and more tolerable labour, and regain their lost figures rapidly. They have a more positive outlook, with less vomiting and food faddism. They are less prone to depression after delivery. This also positively impacts on the baby's health. Babies born to active women are thinner, healthier and less prone to obesity and other metabolic disorders like diabetes and hypertension in later life.

If only parents had their priorities right, we could read matrimonial advertisements saying "educated, employed, healthy, physically fit girl who comes with her own treadmill!"

Chapter 36

Memory Improvement Starts in the Womb

Preparation for public exams have to start really early in today's competitive world. By the time children reach the plus two level it is already too late. Some tuitions and intensive coaching classes start soon after the 8th standard, others after 10th with a last nerve-wracking spurt in the 12th.

To really ensure success, preparation probably has to start from the womb itself.

Families should look after their little girls well, nurturing them physically and mentally, as they are the torchbearers for the next generation. Girls should be provided with a diet adequate in calories and minerals, especially iron and calcium so that they grow strong.

Folic acid supplements should be started soon after menarche so that there are sufficient body stores for the brain development of the next generation. Girls should be encouraged to be physically active so that pregnancy is stress and complication free, the delivery normal, and lactation established and sufficient. The incidence of depression after delivery is also reduced. This means the child receives better nurturing.

In order maximize the unborn child's intelligence

> The mother should have finished high school and be at least twenty years old.

> Pregnancies should be planned, even in arranged marriages, so that only 1 or 2 spaced and wanted children are born.

> Financial security and should be achieved with a good job and steady income, before starting a family as rearing children is expensive.

A pregnant woman

➢ Should receive adequate balanced nutrition.

➢ Exercise regularly.

➢ Avoid stress.

➢ Read aloud to the unborn baby, recite mathematical tables and listen to classical music. All this stimulates the unborn baby's brain cells while still inside the uterus, and has a beneficial effect.

Between 50% and 80 % of a child's intelligence is inherited from the parents. Children are born with 12 billion brain cells. Neurons (brain cells) that are not used by the time the child is twelve years old die irrevocably, until only around 6 billion neurons survive in adult life. Parents can nurture and stimulate inherited intelligence to retain brain cells, and realize its full potential.

Time spent with the baby stimulates it, and arouses curiosity. Nurturing with love without harsh physical discipline helps in developing emotional intelligence, essential for a successful career.

The first two years of life are the most important for the growing brain. New neuron connections are made as the baby is exposed to new sights, sounds, odours, and tastes. Children should be stimulated to explore the world around them. Listening to classical music and being read aloud to increases inherited intelligence by a few points. Since their understanding is limited and their attention span short, their curiosity should be aroused without over stimulation.

Children require playing to learn to adapt. By playing with real objects, they learn where how and why things work. This inculcates the art of logic and reasoning which holds them in good stead in examinations in later life.

After birth, exclusive breast feeding until the age of 4–6 months is best for the baby's brain development. It contains everything (including omega 3 fatty acids) in the correct proportions.

Toddlers should be provided with a diet containing sufficient protein. The habit of eating breakfast should be taught early so that it continues through the school years. This gives the brain a jump-start in the morning.

A child's memory bank can be built and stimulated to enhance their language and mathematical skills. Memory can be stimulated by

- ➤ Established routines. Children love order and even very young children can eagerly anticipate and remember "what comes next?" A chaotic unstructured existence fails to establish brain pathways.

- ➤ Reinforce memory by asking questions like "who is this? What is this?"

- ➤ Imitation should be encouraged. Instead of doing something for the child encourage the child to follow your actions. Learning will be faster and more pleasurable

- ➤ School going children should have their brain stimulated with jigsaw puzzles, word games, and three dimensional puzzles like the Rubick's cube and some traditional Indian, Japanese and Chinese puzzles, not cartoon network and TV serials.

- ➤ Adequate protein at breakfast and lunch helps the brain learn and retain in school.

- ➤ Physical activity helps in the oxygenation and efficient activity of the brain tissue.

- ➤ Playing does not mean sitting in the house alone with toys. It means running, climbing, swinging and interaction with peers.

Parents need to lead by example. Hard work and studying are habits essential for success which cannot really be taught. They are learnt and entrenched from childhood by observation of adults in the environment. Inherently intelligent children receive a boost when they have interested and motivated parents. Slow learners usually have hidden talents in other areas waiting to be recognized and developed. Academic underperformance may be offset by talent in the fine arts or sports.

Encouragement and reinforcement go a long way to helping every child realize their full potential.

Better children for a brighter tomorrow.

Chapter 37

"Sex Scans and Scams"

"Is my baby a boy or a girl? I already have one girl. I do not want another one."

Unhappy, tense, the woman rarely says, "Is my second child normal?"

In this is era of small families, the latter is a more legitimate question.

The answer is that no one can really guarantee a normal outcome for any pregnancy, but the odds can reduced if you do not have any risk factors like , consanguinity, a previously abnormal baby, a genetic defect or any illnesses or complications during pregnancy.

Besides, without resorting to any scientific procedure, anyone predicting the sex of a baby will be correct 50 % of the time as the choices is only male or female! This gives a lot of room for quacks, fortune tellers, soothsayers and other charlatans to make a fast buck. Some even offer a money-back guarantee if they are wrong!

Every Indian woman has the right to choose the number of children she wants to have, one, two or more. She can opt for contraception or terminate an unwanted pregnancy. Under the provisions of the medical termination of pregnancy act, there are many reasons for legal termination, like failure of contraception or mental ill-health. It is however illegal to terminate a pregnancy just because you are not satisfied with the sex of the baby and would have preferred something else..

Prenatal (prior to birth) genetic testing and sex determination is legally offered to couples with a family history of a known disorder based on family history, maternal age and history of previous bad obstetric outcome. Eligible couples usually have already had a previous affected infant, with thalassaemia, sickle cell disease, X linked congenital diseases like Duchenne and Becker muscular dystrophy, fragile Xsyndrome or hemophilia.

X linked diseases solely affect the male child, as he receives a X chromosome from his mother carrying the defective gene. He receives a Y from the father, so that any genetic defect on the X is expressed. His sister on the other hand is spared as she has an abnormal X from her mother and this is over ridden by the normal X from the father. In short, the boy is affected and the girl is a carrier of the disease. In this scenario, it is the affected male baby that is terminated.

To determine if the baby is normal, an ultrasound scan is a safe non-invasive technique. If performed around the 18 – 20 week, it can pick up positions of the baby, determine the age, diagnose multiple pregnancy (twins or triplets), skeletal abnormalities, hydrocephalus, anencephaly, polydactyly,(multiple fingers and toes) the structure of the face, heart, gastrointestinal tract and kidneys. It can also determine the sex of the baby with some degree of accuracy.

The machine itself cannot interpret the images, so a correct report has to come from an experienced trained qualified sonologist.

Chorionic villi sampling can performed under ultrasound guidance, by aspirating some of the cells from the placenta inside the uterus at 10–12 weeks gestation. It is used for karyotyping and determining the foetal sex.

Amniocentesis is done by aspirating a small quantity of amniotic fluid from the uterus at 14–15 weeks. It is used for the diagnosis of chromosomal and genetic disorders, determining the foetal sex, assessing foetal maturity (if done close to the date of delivery), diagnosing some genetically transmitted inborn errors of metabolism, and for brain and spinal cord defects.

Amniocentesis and chorionic villi sampling are specialized procedures. They should be undertaken for diagnostic purposes by academically oriented qualified obstetricians with access to a competent laboratory capable of accurate interpretation of the samples provided.

Unfortunately, in India today, there is a total disregard for medical and legal guidelines. Preying on the Indian psyche with its penchant for the male child, prenatal sexing and abortion of the healthy, but unwanted financially burdensome female foetus is widely practiced.

Also, accurate sexing can be done only in the second trimester, when abortions are dangerous.

This practice is a striking example of rampant misuse of advances in science and technology.

Female feticide (abortion) is illegal. The law punishes the doctor, the relatives and the mother with fines and imprisonment.

This is not a deterrent, as the medical termination of an unwanted unsexed pregnancy itself is not illegal. This leaves a large loophole in the law for female feticide, with the connivance of all the concerned parties and the wilful absence of documentation. There is no conversation only sign language to expose the sex of the unborn child. Code words are used like "the sky is blue." Women are their own enemies, as aborting the female foetus is done with the connivance of the mother, and grandmother with the assistance of an unprincipled medical practitioner.

Fly by night operators tapping a vulnerable market offer these services. The threat of imprisonment makes the fees high both for the determination and for the termination. The bottom lime is money, an effort to earn income they are probably not competent enough to earn legally, with a total disregard for the social and demographic consequences of such actions.

Illegal sex determination has gone high tech with portable ultrasound machines, and mobile operating theatres in vans with generators. These go out into the villages and offer these illegal services.

The slogan is simple and direct.

Pay 500 today determine the sex. Pay 5000 tomorrow abort the unwanted female child or refuse the offer at your own peril and pay upwards of 500000 for the marriage expenses.

Women, in a placatory, docile, non-confrontational attempt to produce the required number of male progeny, wind up undergoing repeated surgical terminations. More than half confessed that the husband and his family had coerced them into the procedure. Refusal to comply could result in infanticide, with the girls choked or suffocated to death. Mothers found this more unbearable to witness and preferred an abortion. Sometimes the husband threatened to remarry a more docile woman in an attempt to produce an heir.

Repeated abortions affect the mother's general and reproductive health. She may eventually be unable to carry a pregnancy of the right sex to term.

Today, approximately fifty million women are "missing" in the Indian population. Remember, one of them might even our next president!

In most countries in the world, there are approximately 105 female births for every 100 males. In India, there are less than 93 women for every 100 men in the population. The accepted reason for such a disparity is the practice of female infanticide in India, especially in urban and rural North / Northwest states, and urban parts of some Central and Western states.

Despite overall mortality decline, child mortality is also greater among girls than boys. Female child mortality is due to selective neglect and female infanticide.

Medical practitioners advertise and perform prenatal sex determination tests without using their judgment. They are not coerced. They do not reflect about the moral and ethical aspects of their actions or the consequences of rampant commercial sex determination. They do the tests and the terminations purely for the sake of money. In the process, they increase sexual discrimination and exploitation of women in society.

Watch out! Think! We are heading for a dangerous surplus of males! Our sons need mates! Where are they going to find them?

CHAPTER 38

CONTRACEPTION

Postponing—spacing—finishing! Should we recklessly "go forth and procreate?"

Indian women theoretically have the freedom to determine the size of their families and the spacing of their children. The government provides free contraceptive methods to suit every budget, age group and family size. Husbands and mother's in law no longer have to consent to any method of contraception, temporary or permanent chosen by the woman. It is also illegal to divorce a woman or practice polygamy if the wife fails to produce the requisite number of progeny of the correct sex.

However, the scenario in the "real India" is different. Sex education is not a compulsory part of our school curriculum. "Arranged" marriages are still the norm. Alliances between families are arranged by marriage brokers, relatives, friends and well-wishers. Everyone wants to see the girl "settled." These brides are often barely out of their teens. They enter matrimony with inaccurate and inadequate knowledge of contraception gained from "old wives tales" and married peers. The bride, mentally and physically unprepared to face the challenges of mother hood, unfortunately lacks the knowledge to delay the inevitable.

At present, 1027 million married Indian women (16% of the total) have unmet contraceptive needs. They are unable to space their families (30 %) or to stop procreation (86%).

In addition, 15–30 % of unmarried boys and 10 % of unmarried girls are engaged in unprotected high-risk sexually active behaviour. Failure to prevent unwanted pregnancies results in psychological problems, forced marriages and clandestine abortions. Being an unwed single mother is still not a viable option in India.

Several options are available for contraception. The method eventually chosen depends on motivation, adequate information, an individual's requirements and on available medical support.

The methods can be divided into two main groups, the ones dependent on the individual woman alone, or those also requiring male cooperation.

Oral contraceptive pills (OCPs) contain oestrogen and progesterone. They are a safe and efficient method, whose success depends only on the motivated woman alone. The pills can be consumed openly or clandestinely, and can be taken for as long as desired. They have to be taken at the same time every day, irrespective of changing meal timings or fasting. There may be a few mild side effects, which tend to disappear as the pills are continued. Otherwise, switching brands may do the trick, as the ratio of the hormones as well as the particular derivatives used differ from one manufacturer to another.

Oral contraceptive pills can be purchased in pharmacies or picked up free at government-authorized family planning out lets. They are packaged as 21 or 28 tablets. The active ingredient is present in 21 tablets and the remaining 7 have inactive ingredients to preserve continuity in the "pill popping" habit.

ONCE STARTED, they should be taken REGULARLY at THE SAME TIME, preferably at night. In the 21 tablet formulations, the tablets are consumed for 21days and stopped for 7, (three weeks on and one week off). Medication is taken strictly according to the calendar, and NOT ACCORDING TO THE MENUSTRAL CYCLE, or the timing of intercourse. Taking a pill only when you have sex will not protect you.

In the 28 tablet packs there is no break.

If a tablet is forgotten then two can be taken the next day at 12-hour intervals (morning and evening). If more than 2 tablets are missed (2 days) there is no protection against pregnancy.

Stopping the pill reverses its effects and pregnancy usually soon follows within a few cycles.

OCPs do not cause cancer of the ovary or uterus or permanent sterility.

Contraindications to its use are smoking, carcinoma of the breast, recurrent blood clots, bleeding into the brain or liver disease.

Progesterone only pills are available for use during lactation and in women who are unable to tolerate oestrogen preparations. They have to be taken continuously (no break).

Women who unwilling to swallow tablets regularly can opt for long acting "depo" injections of progesterone.. Depending on the formulation they are administered once in 2 months (8 weeks norethisterone) or 3 months(12 weeks) medroxyprogesterone).

Alternatively intrauterine devices can be used. The Government provides the "copper T" free. Similar devices like the Cu 250 or 350, can be purchased from pharmacies. They need to be inserted and removed by qualified personnel. It is technically easier to insert them during menstruation. They can be left in place for periods ranging from 3–5 years depending on the type of device. A small percentage of women (0.1%) can conceive with the copper T in place. Sometimes, such a pregnancy can occur in the fallopian tubes. If you miss a period please check with the doctor and do a pregnancy test.

Diaphragms and female condoms are cumbersome and unpopular in India.

Less effective methods are pessaries, jellies and spermicidal creams.

"Male dependent" methods succeed with a motivated, cooperative and responsible partner. One out of ten couples in India successfully practices "natural methods" like total abstinence (no sex). This is difficult as there is a biological need in most men. Others practice "coitus interruptus" (ejaculation outside the vagina). This is requires motivation and control.

In the "rhythm" method intercourse is confined to the "safe period." This can be calculated if the woman has a regular menstrual cycle (usually ranging from 26 to 32 days). Intercourse is confined to the 9 days BEFORE menstruation, the 4 days DURING menstruation and three days AFTER. A simple way to calculate this is to AVOID intercourse from days 8 to 19, the first day of bleeding being day 1.

If the woman's cycle is irregular this calculation and method is doomed to failure.

Condoms are provided free in family planning clinics. They are popular and can also be purchased in road side shops, supermarkets or pharmacies. They should be put on after erection and before penetration and ejaculation. They should be disposed off hygienically. Condoms are NOT washable or reusable. They protect against unwanted pregnancy and sexual transmitted diseases like gonorrhoea, syphilis, Chlamydia, herpes and AIDS.

Emergency contraception is available and effective if taken within 72 hours of unprotected intercourse, NOT 72 hours after a missed period. The "Yuzpe" regimen or levonorgesterol alone can be used in the correct protocol. If frequent recourse to emergency contraception is required then it is more sensible to opt for a regular long-term method.

The above methods are reversible.

After the age of 35, or if either partner feels their family is complete and they do not want any more children, a permanent method like tubectomy in the female or vasectomy in the male. It should be seriously considered as an option. This removes the stress and fear of an unwanted pregnancy late in life, when the other children are grown up.

During the reproductive age group, when contraception is being used, regular evaluation of reproductive health of the woman should be done at 6-month intervals. At any time if there is a delay in the onset of the menstruation, a prompt evaluation for "contraceptive failure" resulting in pregnancy should be done. A non-invasive urine test is usually sufficient.

If the inevitable has occurred, do not panic, consult your physician as there are several safe options available. The friendly neighbourhood pharmacist with "Mensoon and Mensovit are not the solution!

Medical options are available for terminating an unwanted pregnancy safely up to the 49 th day. A combination of mifepristone, or methotrexate and misoprostol can be used in the correct dose under medical supervision, for a medical termination. These are not OTC drugs and cannot be dispensed without a prescription.

Surgical procedures for termination of an unwanted pregnancy up to 20 weeks is legal under the provisions of the MTP act passed in 1971. They are not clandestine or illegal. They are free in government hospitals.

To avoid the misuse of induced abortions the Medical Termination of Pregnancy Act was enacted by the Indian Parliament in 1971 and revised again in 1975. The MTP Act lays down the condition under which a pregnancy can be terminated, the persons and the place to perform it.

The reasons, for which MTP is done, as interpreted from the Indian MTP Act, are:

i. Where a pregnant woman has a serious medical disease and continuation of pregnancy could endanger her life like: Heart diseases, severe rise in blood pressure, uncontrolled vomiting during pregnancy, cancer of the breast or cervix, diabetes mellitus with eye complication (retinopathy), epilepsy or psychiatric illness.

ii. Where the continuation of pregnancy could lead to substantial risk to the newborn leading to serious physical / mental handicaps examples like chromosomal abnormalities, rubella (German measles), viral infections in the mother in first three months, if previous children have congenital abnormalities, Rh iso-immunisation. exposure of the foetus to irradiation.

iii. Pregnancy resulting of rape.

iv. Conditions where the socio-economic status of the mother (family) hampers the progress of a healthy pregnancy and the birth of a healthy child.

v. Failure of Contraceptive Device irrespective of the method used (natural methods/ barrier methods/ hormonal methods). This condition is a unique feature of the Indian Law. All the pregnancies can be terminated using this criterion.

Consent:

If married— her own written consent. Husband's consent not required.

If unmarried and above 18years —her own written consent.

If below 18 years —written consent of her guardian.

If mentally unstable — written consent of her guardian.

A signed consent assures the clinician performing the abortion that the woman has been informed of all her options, has been counselled about the procedure, its risks and how to care for herself after she chosen the abortion of her own free will.

Lack of knowledge, results in approximately 6–7 million dangerous illegal abortions being performed a year. Many of these are performed by quacks and endanger the life of the mother. There is no need for this as the government by passing the MTP act has ensured safety confidentiality and free choice.

Contraception is a very personal and confidential matter. It should be offered without prejudice to the reproductive age group. Couples provided with adequate information should be able to say with confidence "we know when, why, and how!"

CHAPTER 39

MENOPAUSE

The woman was seated alone in a corner of the mixed bar from the time it opened at 11 am. She sat silently and steadfastly puffed pack after pack of cigarettes and downed gins one after another. This was not London Paris or New York, but urban India.

Lonely menopausal women, with an empty nest, drinking publicly, is common sight in the west, but still rare in India. Now with globalization, cultures are obviously changing.

Menopause or the climacteric is the cessation of menstruation and is diagnosed if no bleeding has occurred for a period of 12 months. It marks an end to the reproductive phase of the woman's life.

Our grandmothers died young, but today, women spend as much as half their life after menopause. Their children are grown up and gone and their work load is less. Many have never been encouraged to take up a career. Now suddenly it seems too late, and life seems to have passed them by.

Menstruation is under the control of several hormones, released by the pituitary and hypothalamus in the brain and the ovaries. These hormones do not cease to function overnight. Instead, the release of the hormones become erratic and this imbalance gives rise to many of the symptoms of menopause.

After surgery involving hysterectomy and oopherectomy (removal of the uterus and ovaries), menopause occurs abruptly and is more severe than in natural menopause.

The age at which menopause begins varies. Some women reach menopause in their 30s or 40s, and some not until they are nearly 60, but menopause most often occurs between the ages of 45 and 55.

Some lucky women have no symptoms at all and breeze through their menopause. Others find it a long and arduous journey on rocky unfamiliar terrain.

The first indication or perimenopause signalling that menopause is approaching is menstrual irregularities; the unbalanced hormone levels cause them to become unpredictable. They become more frequent or the intervals become longer. There are no longer any safe days, as sudden torrential bleeding may occur in the embarrassing circumstances. As the hormones are not perfectly balanced, sometimes the periods become infrequent and scanty. Contraception should be continued until menstruation has ceased for a full year as egg release though erratic does occur and pregnancy can result.

Oestrogen levels fall and FSH (follicle stimulating hormone) levels rise. This makes the superficial blood vessels in the skin expand leading to warmth, flushing, blushing, sweating and chills. The sudden flushing may cause the skin in fair women to turn an angry red. This is followed by profuse drenching sweats. Professional women find this embarrassing as it may occur several times during the day. When they occur at night, they disturb sleep, leading to insomnia, fatigue, depression and stress.

The physical appearance may change subtly. The relative increase in male hormone changes the texture of the skin, and may produce acne and facial hair. A moustache and side burns maybe unsightly. The slowing metabolism causes loss of muscle strength and an increase in weight. The shoulders broaden a paunch appears and arms become flabby.

Oestrogen influences the mental well being of the patient. Inadequate levels cause irritability, fatigue, decreased memory and diminished concentration. A previously alert and happy woman may feel depressed and disoriented. She may forget things, names, numbers and details.

Women are protected by hormones to some extent against heart disease. With this gone their incidence of heart disease equals that of men. Heart attacks become a common cause of death.

The bone density reduces at a rapid rate, increasing the risk of osteoporosis. The bones to become brittle and weak, and there is an increased risk of fractures, especially of the hip spine and wrist. There may be a stooped and bent appearance and a reduction in height as the vertebral bodies collapse on each other.

The tissues of the vagina and urethra lose their elasticity. This gives rise to frequency, urgency or even more embarrassing, incontinence with coughing, sneezing or laughing. Sex may become painful.

Most of these problems can be tackled with a knowledge and motivation.

➤ Reduce the quantity of food eaten by 1 iddly or chappati. Do not take a second helping

➤ Exercise regularly. Instead of the bare minimum of 30 minutes 4 days a week, try to go faster and longer to compensate for the slowing metabolism.

➤ Do weight training exercises using "baby dumbbells." A half kilo weight and twenty repetitions is sufficient.

➤ A hairy appearance can be tackled by regular visits to the beauty parlour.

➤ Hot flashes usually have a trigger which sets them off, like hot tea or coffee and spicy food. Avoid the triggers and dress in light airy clothing.

➤ Vaginal dryness and discomfort can be tackled with water-based lubricants like K-Y Jelly, or moisturizers like Vaseline or vaginal oestrogen creams.

➤ Pelvic floor muscle exercises, (Kegel exercises), improve urinary incontinence. At least 3 times a day concentrate on the muscles required to stop urination in mid stream and tighten them. Repeat 20 times.

➤ Build up bone density with regular calcium (1200mg/day). Assimilation into the bone can be helped if necessary with alendrolate or the SERMS group of medications. However though calcium can be continued life lon, alendrolate should be stopped after 3 years.

➢ Schedule regular medical check ups for mammograms, Pap tests, and lipid level (cholesterol and triglyceride) testing. Mammograms usually need to be repeated every 3 years. Sometimes the doctor may feel that an ultrasound of the breast is sufficient. The frequency of the Pap test depends on whether any abnormality was detected the first time. Cholesterol, triglycerides and sugars should be checked every 6 months to a year.

➢ Do not smoke.

Some patients benefit from a short course of hormone replacement therapy (HRT) to tide them over intolerable symptoms. This consists of a small dose of natural oestrogen combined with progesterone in women who have an intact uterus. Oestrogen is given alone if the uterus has been surgically removed. HRT has generated a lot of controversy. Initially pushed as the "magic bullet" for all menopausal ailments, it now has fallen into disrepute because of side effects. One of the company's manufacturing this medication has now closed down. It is beneficial in a small number of women for a few months for uncontrollable intolerable hot flashes.

There are natural phytoestrogens, in soya and yam. Initially they were extensively propagated and may help but should not be taken by women who have a family history of breast cancer or abnormal mammograms. Evening primrose oil capsules or vitamin E (less than 400 IU) may be beneficial, but their effects are not scientifically proven. Some women require low-dose antidepressants to help them cope.

A year later, the woman was seated in the same place at same time puffing and drinking. She looked older, more depressed and had become stooped and bent. A wasted life, with at least twenty years more in the same situation!

Life after menopause does not have to be like that. It can be healthy meaningful and fulfilling.

Chapter 40

Stress Incontinence

Women cook, clean, produce children, and often cope with the additional physical and emotional demands of a profession or job. As they grow older, an expanding waistline, the stress of reproduction and the hormonal changes of menopause take their toll. Activities like coughing, sneezing, laughing, exercising, cause a few drops of urine to involuntarily escape even though the bladder is not full.

Multiple vaginal births increase the risk of stress incontinence as the pelvic musculature is weakened or damaged. Menopause decreases the female hormones, causing atrophy of the vagina and loss of pelvic muscle tone. Both cause the bladder to protrude into the vaginal space increasing incontinence,

50% of all women have occasional urinary incontinence and 10% have frequent incontinence. The incidence increases until 20% of women over age 75 experience daily urinary incontinence.

Urinary incontinence does not exclusively affect women. Affected males usually have a correctable underlying precipitating factor like an enlarged prostate, a BMI more than 30, or chronic bronchitis. Both obesity and chronic cough increases the incidence. Incontinence is also commoner in smokers and asthmatics.

Pelvic surgery can inadvertently damage the nerves supplying the bladder producing stress incontinence in a previously normal individual.

Stress incontinence is different from "urge incontinence" when a strong desire to urinate escapes voluntary control. The bladder precipitously empties partially or completely en route to the toilet.

An urge to void occurs when the bladder contains 200 ml of urine. It can stretch to accommodate 500ml. In "over flow" incontinence urine escapes in small quantities from a full bladder.

Urine stains are visible on light coloured clothing causing social embarrassment.. Repeated episodes cause soreness of the external genitalia. A faint smell of urine may emanate from the affected individual.

Can anything be more awkward?

Eventually, the person can become self-conscious, diffident, withdrawn and a social outcast.

Once stress incontinence has been clinically diagnosed, a few basic tests should be done.

- ➢ A physical pelvic examination to rule out abnormalities of the pelvic organs.
- ➢ Blood tests to rule out diabetes.
- ➢ Urinalysis and culture if infection is suspected.
- ➢ A few simple life style interventions can help to reduce stress incontinence.
- ➢ Reduction in weight so that the BMI (body mass index) is around 25.
- ➢ Control over volume of fluids drunk and reduction in the quantity if it is more than 2–3 litres/day.
- ➢ Prevention of constipation as hard faecal matter acts as an obstruction and aggravates stress incontinence.
- ➢ Regular voiding, so that the bladder is never too full.

Women can retrain pelvic muscles, which voluntarily control urination, and regain lost tone by performing Kegel exercises regularly. These help strengthen the muscles of the pelvic floor, and improve the urethral sphincter function. The muscles should be consciously contracted for a count of 20, 15 times twice a day. To ensure the correct muscles are being used, try to stop the urine stream in mid flow. Alternatively each time you go to the toilet to pass urine, stop and restart the process voluntarily several times, so that you exert control over the action. Within 4 weeks, 70% of women markedly improve and 15 % are permanently cured. The benefit disappears within a few days if the exercises are not consciously continued.

Tricyclic antidepressants and other medications can be used to treat stress incontinence in patients with mild-to-moderate symptoms. 50 % of the people respond favourably.

Oestrogen replacement, either taken orally as part of HRT (hormone replacement therapy), or applied locally in the vagina as a cream improves urinary frequency, urgency, stress incontinence and burning in postmenopausal women.

Surgical treatment can be considered after a thorough evaluation, examination and investigation to determination of the exact cause of the urinary incontinence. Surgery can help by correcting the anatomical abnormalities. The bladder and urethra are supported in the proper position, and the urethral sphincter tightened. This helps achieve voluntary control. Surgery has a 75% to 95% cure rate if the patients are carefully selected. The procedure involves anaesthesia and hospital stay and is not totally risk free..

The eventual outcome is unsatisfactory in people:

➤ With prior surgical failures.

➤ If there are other genital or urinary problems

➤ Or other complicating diseases that may prevent adequate healing or make the technical aspects of the surgery more difficult.

As age advances, the bladder capacity reduces; the urinary stream becomes weaker, and visits to the toilet more frequent. This does not mean that urinary frequency, urgency and stress incontinence have to be accepted as an inevitable part of aging. The bladder can be re-trained by consciously increasing the time between voiding. Adherence to Keegle's exercises can result is a "cure" as long as the schedule is maintained.

Most incontinence problems, provided they do not require corrective surgery, can be cured by motivation, weight loss and pelvic exercises.

Chapter 41

Andropause, a Male Mid-Life Crisis

Older men sometimes go to physicians complaining that their bodies no longer obey mental commands with precision and speed. In addition, they snore, have sleep disturbances, memory loss and weight gain. A few express more embarrassing complaints like a low sex drive, enlarging breasts and difficulty in passing urine. If accompanied by a partner or caretaker other unexpressed symptoms emerge, like grumpiness, irritability, emotional changes and loss of libido.

These changes are accepted in older women. They appear close to menopause, when falling oestrogen levels can be documented. Physicians often fail to recognize a similar stage in older men.

Society expects men to be stoic and macho with no hint of weakness. Also, these symptoms can coincide with other changes and upheavals in the man's life, suggesting a co-existing underlying depression.

Andropause is often considered a myth. Many symptoms are subjective, but a physical examination can reveal decreased muscle mass, reduced strength and increased fat deposits. The shoulders may be rounded and the height decreased with weak and osteoporotic bones.

The rise and fall of hormone levels in men is gradual, subtle and less well documented in men than in women. The diagnosis is often clinical

Testosterone (male hormone) assays have only now become sensitive and reliable. Total testosterone, is low only in a fifth of cases. The available testosterone, the free androgen index (FAI) is decreased in three quarters of cases, but this can be demonstrated only by sophisticated and expensive blood analyses.

The quality of life that a man leads is affected by the fall in the level of testosterone. Many disease processes are aggravated and accelerated.

- ➤ Osteoporosis, though commoner in women, can occur in men as the testosterone levels fall. The male bone density normally falls between 40 and 70 years. One fifth of men over age 50 actually have osteoporosis, putting then at risk of fractures of the wrists, hips, spine and ribs.

- ➤ There is also an association between low-testosterone levels and an increased risk of heart attacks.

Early treatments for the male menopause were offered clandestinely in men's magazines, trains and bus stations. They focussed only on the falling sex drive. Dubious fly-by-night operators advertised remedies like monkey-gland extract, powdered rhinoceros horn or Spanish fly. These were and consumed by unsuspecting individuals. Sometimes heavy metals like gold were administered in dangerous and toxic doses.

Initially, physicians did not take andropause seriously. HRT (Hormone Replacement Therapy) was being advocated as the magic bullet to overcome the distressing effects of loss of estrogens at menopause, for women. In the same way, carefully monitored Testosterone Replacement Therapy (TRT) has been advocated for men.

It is less popular; even though it probably does slow the "ageing" process in men. Titration and dosing are more difficult. There is no clear indication of exactly who would benefit. Acceleration of undetected cancer of the prostate is a very real fear. Earlier forms of oral testosterone were toxic to the liver. Injections were painful. Despite benefits, and careful selection of patients it is not very popular.

Now, a great deal of research has gone into the development of masculinity preserving medication to put "the man back into manhood". It has generated more interest and funding than other commoner issues in geriatric research. Widely publicized sidenofil citrate (Viagra) was discovered, "a giant performance leap for mankind".

Yet, many men today do not want to admit that they have a problem. Desperately, clandestinely they resort to purchases of an OTC mixture of Viagra and testosterone. This is dangerous. Viagra can cause sudden death in embarrassing situations in heart patients, particularly in those already on medication. Contrary to widely circulated stories, it does not prolong the organism nor heighten desire in a psychologically unprepared male. It is better to seek expert help for sexual dysfunctions.

ADAM (Androgen Decline in Aging Males) alone may not be responsible for falling hormone levels.

It can occur in

> In hormonal deficiencies like hypothyroidism, and in pituitary and adrenal tumours.

> In anaemia.

> With obesity when the BMI is over 30 (weight in kg divided by the height in meter squared).

> Chronic regular alcohol consumption.

> Diabetes, especially if it is uncontrolled.

> Liver and kidney diseases.

> Stress.

> Chronic illness.

> Some medications

To turn back the clock of time.

> Maintain ideal body weight. As the rate of body metabolism naturally slows down with age, this means moving faster over longer distances to maintain the same weight.

> Walk or jog 30–40 mins 5–6 days a week.

> Do weight training with light weights. This slows down loss of muscle mass, helps maintain tone and posture, and helps in

the control of diabetes and hypertension. It also helps men to stand straight and walk tall, and promotes an all round sense of well being.

➢ Yoga meditation and prayer will help to relieve stress and provide a focus and meaning to life.

➢ Supplements of calcium will help maintain bone strength.

ADAM can be offset by natural healthy aging.

Don't let hormones control your life!

CHAPTER 42

SNORING

Watch Out! It may be Fatal

Snorers are the butt of jokes. The rhythmic loud buzzing sounds they emit disrupts the sleep of everyone in the vicinity. It is difficult to sleep in an airline or railway compartment surrounded by musical snores of various pitches throughout the night. It is an ingenious form of torture.

No one snores on purpose. Snoring is an involuntary action. Unfortunately, snorers cannot hear themselves. They seldom wake up with the noise they make. They are unwilling to accept accusations of loud noise and disrupted sleep without proof.

Snoring can occur in all ages and both sexes. It is commoner in the older age group, in males and in the overweight. 45% of all adults are occasional snorers and 25 % habitual snorers.

Snoring in adult life is harmful for health. It causes disturbs normal restful sleep patterns and produces sleep deprivation. This in turn causes day time drowsiness, blunts mental capabilities and decision making, and increases stress. Decreased concentration makes driving and operating machinery difficult. The person may become accident prone.

People who snore also tend to develop high blood pressure and suffer from heart attacks. This may because obese persons tend to snore. Obesity itself is an independent risk factor for hypertension and heart disease.

The sudden onset of snoring in a previously healthy person needs to be evaluated. It may be due to the appearance of a benign or malignant tumour in the nose or throat.

Children snore if they have large tonsils and adenoids which cause internal narrowing and obstruction of the airways. If the snoring child is also a habitual mouth breather, or has recurrent attacks of tonsillitis then a qualified ENT surgeon may advice surgical removal of the tonsils and adenoids. This decision should not be made lightly as tonsils are not "useless " They are the body's first line of defence against respiratory infections.

Sometimes, allergies or a cold may cause a temporary swelling of the nasal passages. The obstruction may create an exaggerated vacuum in the throat during breathing and this produces a snore. Treatment of the cold cures the snoring.

Habitual snorers have less space between the tongue and soft palate. The tissues then strike each other and vibrate during breathing. This may be because of an abnormally long soft palate. It dangles loosely making a noise as air moves in and out. Sometimes deformities of the nose, such as a deviated septum can cause an obstruction while breathing and produce snoring. In an overweight person, the thick neck can cause obstruction from outside and snoring. Weakness or paralysis of the palatal muscles can cause them to move loosely while breathing producing loud sounds. This can occur with increasing age.

Consumption of alcohol, tranquilizers or sedatives can cause excessive relaxation of the muscles used for breathing. This can also produce a noise.

Sometimes, loud snoring is interspersed with episodes of no breathing at all. This is called obstructive sleep apnoea. It usually lasts for10 seconds and occurs several times during the night. This reduces blood oxygen levels. The person sleeps lightly and fitfully, keeping his muscles tense and his mind alert. The heart reacts by pumping harder and faster. Eventually the sufferer evolves into an obese stressed out sleep deprived hypertensive.

There are a number of devices on the market to reduce snoring. Some of them do work, but this may be because they also prevent deep sleep, when snoring is most likely to occur.

A rubber ball can be sewn on to the back of the night shirt. This prevents the person from sleeping on his back and reduces snoring. The person can use pillows to sleep on one side as lying flat increases the snoring.

There are some exercises to strengthen the palate and neck muscles. Press your head downwards while you try to force the chin upwards with your hand. Place both fingers in the ears and make an "aah" sound.

Snoring may respond to various surgical procedures. Ablation and tightening may be done using heat, radio waves or lasers or with conventional surgery. These tighten flabby tissues in the throat and palate, and expand air passages. More or less the same result can be medically obtained by using a nasal mask that delivers air under pressure into the throat. This has to be used every night and is called continuous positive airway pressure or "CPAP".

Also,

➢ Adopt a healthy lifestyle.

➢ Develop good muscle tone with regular exercise.

➢ Maintain an ideal body weight.

➢ Avoid tranquilizers, sleeping pills, and antihistamines before bedtime.

➢ Avoid alcohol and heavy meals for three hours before sleeping.

➢ Sleep sufficiently at regular hours.

➢ Sleep on one side not on your back.

➢ Snoring indicates an airway obstruction that is serious, not hopeless or funny.

A woman was in the news for having smothered and then stabbed her husband. Asked why, she replied, "he snored." Don't let the same fate befall you!

CHAPTER 43

WEANING

Feeding and Successful weaning – a d(r)ying art?

The child looked with great interest at the array of plastic feeding bottles on the counter and asked, "If all ammas have two feeding bottles fixed to their chests, then, why are these plastic bottles sold in shops?"

A pertinent question in today's world! After all, there seem to be unsatisfactory instant solutions for everything, including breast feeding and weaning.

Female mammals differ from other animals in that they have breast milk for their babies, which is initially sufficient. After a certain period of time, as the baby matures and grows it has to be weaned from the breast and started on a solid diet. This is accomplished effortlessly in lower animals. In humans, weaning is a drawn out, tension producing, emotionally demanding, frustrating and sometimes unsuccessful process.

The WHO has stated that weaning should be started no earlier than the 4th month (120 days). Until then exclusive breast feeding (no supplements including water) are required.

If the baby is happy after the breast feed, not crying, and is gaining weight at a satisfactory rate then weaning can be delayed to the 6th month. A child who is constantly hungry and not gaining weight in an upward curve needs to be weaned earlier.

Breast milk is bland so the initial weaning food offered should taste similar. Rice or a mixture of rice and ragi can be powdered at home in a food processor. It is then partially cooked in water. Sugar is then added to taste and the cooking is completed in cow's milk. The final product should have the consistency of idly or dosai dough to which a little too much water has been added.

A single feed should initially be offered in the morning. The baby should be placed on the lap in an upright position and the conjee offered with a sterilized (boiled for 10 mins) spoon. The baby may spit. This is because its nervous system has not yet adapted to the idea of swallowing. If the baby refuses, turns its head away or cries, do not persist. Try again the next day at the same time, till a routine is successfully established. After two weeks, a second similar feed can be offered in the evening.

New foods should be introduced only every two weeks. Mashed banana, stewed apple, and freshly prepared orange or musambi juice are easily digested. The yellow "Kerala" banana boiled and mashed can be served alone or with a little sugar. Homemade iddiappam or idly can be served with milk rice and sugar. A mixture of dhals can be cooked with salt, mashed, boiled again and added to mashed rice, boiled potato, carrot or idly.

Slowly a little garlic and pinch or turmeric can be added to the rice and dhals. After 9–10 months, boiled minced chicken or fish can be given.

If there is a family history of allergy it is better to delay the introduction of egg until the age of two.

After the age of 10 months, undiluted cow's milk can be offered in a cup at 10 am and 4 pm. The total quantity per day should not exceed 500 ml.

Through all this breast feeding should be continued. As the weaning progresses, and the demand for breast milk decreases, the milk supply will automatically fall. Eventually, at the end of a year when the weaning is complete, the breasts automatically stop production, do not become engorged and are unlikely to develop infections.

Travel becomes easy if the child gets used to eating bananas. They are available everywhere and are sterile if the skin is intact.

All mammals are different. Females successfully produce milk with the composition most suited to their species. Substituting solid weaning foods with milk of other mammals like cows, goats, buffaloes, or donkeys is not advisable.

Carbonated colas and other squashes should not be given to babies even though they express an interest in consuming them. They contain artificial colouring matter, chemicals and preservatives. Some may produce allergies. Others are harmful. The caffeine in some colas can produce appetite suppression, lack of sleep and distressing hyperactivity.

Tea and coffee also contain caffeine. It should not be offered to children under the age of 14.

Many packaged ready to eat weaning cereals are sold over the counter. They are widely and slickly advertised in the media. They are overpriced (400 gms costs between Rs 55 and 95). They contain a long list of vitamins, minerals, and trace elements which may not be really necessary. (Most healthy babies only need iron supplements if at all.) If improperly reconstituted, the imbalanced electrolyte composition may actually produce vomiting and can be dangerous.

"Milk biscuits" contain wheat, milk, sugar and fat with chemicals for emulsification, hydrogenation and preservation. It is probably safer and more hygienic to break wheat in a food processor and cook it with oil or ghee, sugar and milk!

My child doesn't eat. I want a tonic. "The request often ends with the distressed mother painstaking recollecting all the unsolicited advice she has received from relatives, friends and other self styled experts and well-wishers.

Translated, without the hype, her statement just means a thin child, who offers no competition weight-wise to a relative's progeny of the same age.

Often weaning has been disorganized, unscheduled and unscientific. Food habits are often faulty, with meals being offered after milk. There is no structured eating schedule or system, with food following the child all over the house.

Tonics, (vitamins, trace elements and minerals) in a syrupy base, cannot really increase anyone's appetite! They are adjuncts and not substitutes for a balanced diet. Slickly packaged appetite stimulants like cyproheptadine are actually potent antihistamines, used for refractory allergy and migraine, with increased appetite as an undesirable side-effect!

Aryuvedic and herbal tonic have ingredients in concentrations which are not yet under the purview of the drug controller. Do you really want to administer those?

Up to the age of four months (120 days) children need breast milk alone, supplied by a caring mother. Breast milk is best, its formulation is totally in sync with your child's growing needs. It is free, uncontaminated and always available on demand.

Some infants are light sleepers and need reassurance and constant proximity to the mother. Restlessness is confused with inadequate feeding, and supplementary bottle feeds offered. Sucking on a rubber nipple required far less effort than feeding on the breast and the infant soon begins to exhibit a preference for the bottle.

A bottle-fed child receives a formula that, despite slick marketing, is still not on par with the "real thing". Every preparation, natural cows milk, skimmed milk, tinned milk has its own drawbacks.

Eventually, babies get into the habit of demanding a bottle at night while dropping off to sleep. While this lessens the burden of the parent, it predisposes the child to "bottle mouth", a cocktail of diseases including dental caries, fungal infections, diarrhoea and ear infections.

At the end of four to six months, a child is usually ready to try solid foods. The birth weight has nearly doubled, there is some amount of head control, a sitting position is possible with support and the baby exhibits interest in food eaten by others.

From this stage onwards, babies exhibit specific likes and dislikes and know when they are full. Spitting, turning the head away and refusal are hints that should be taken.

Initially, food should be in an easily digestible form like broken rice cooked and mashed in milk. If the food is too solid, the baby may choke. The number of feeds can be increased every two weeks. After the age of six months, mashed potatoes, carrots, pulses, bananas and cooked apples can be given. Adding vegetables before fruits may be a good idea as fruits are sweeter and more palatable.

Avoid nuts, toffees, hard sweets and grapes as these may cause choking. A mixed home cooked diet is palatable, calorie rich and rich contains vitamins, minerals and nutrients. Preservatives in tinned and pre-cooked packaged food are harmful.

The birth weight triples at the end of the first year but weight gain slows down after that. After the age of two the weight can be calculated with the formula (Age + 3) x 5 + weight in pounds.

At this time, children eat only small amounts, so frequent feeds (four to six times) should be given. In school going children, meal times (particularly breakfast) should not be a period of stress, with rapid force feeding due to lack of time, impatience, confrontation and sheer futile frustration. All that results is vomiting or a stubborn refusal to eat.

Milk should not be given first thing in the morning as it then suppresses the appetite for the rest of the day. It should be given after breakfast. Caffeine should be avoided. It is found in tea, coffee, cola drinks and chocolate.

If the diet is adequate, with satisfactory weight gain, vitamin supplementation is harmless but not essential. Left to themselves, healthy children adjust adapt and grow. Children are not Maruti cars, rolling off an assembly line, the same standard size and shape.

CHAPTER 44

COLICKY BABIES

My grand father (Indian medical council registration 94) believed in the therapeutic virtues of a little alcohol, (1 oz for adults and a teaspoon for children). He used it for a variety of ailments, most of which began with the letter "I."

Favourites were indigestion, insomnia, intractable pain, incurable illness and irrepressible cough. Allopathic medicine was in its inception, and a shot of alcohol was a good way to "grin and bear it". Unfortunately, we are still doing this today.

Alcohol is added to cough expectorants and appetite stimulating tonics. A constantly replayed advertisement on television shows three generations of smiling mothers all of whom had in camera cured their baby's colic with is a safe, all-natural liquid. It contained ginger, fennel, sodium bicarbonate (baking soda), fructose, and other harmless ingredients. Unfortunately many people miss the fine print, which proclaimed that it also had 4.6 % alcohol. No wonder that the babies and mothers were smiling!

Alarmed by this trend, countries like Canada and Australia have banned the marketing of alcohol containing OTC (over the counter) infant remedies. The Indian government too has banned the addition of alcohol to "anti gripe" mixtures, and now they are labelled "non-alcoholic".

Parents are distressed when their babies cry inconsolably, especially when the sound is loud, long and uncontrolled. The child's face may turn red and the legs may be drawn up to the abdomen. This distressing symptom is called infant colic, and is diagnosed when it appears around 2 weeks of age, 3–4 days a week and lasts for 3ours or longer. It is present in all cultures, both sexes, in bottle and breast fed infants and in primitive tribes where the babies are carried all day.

Parents are depressed by this regular frustrating occurrence. They tend to blame themselves, although, in actual fact it is not a reflection on their parenting skills. These babies are otherwise well fed and gain weight normally.

At the "non colic" times they are pleasant and easy going. The symptoms appear related to faulty digestion and may be partially relieved by burping. In actual fact, indigestion has nothing to do with the pain. The appearance of the colic is also independent of constituents in the mother's diet. Changes in the food do not offer any lasting benefit.

Another theory is that the baby's immature nervous system is unable to come to terms with the rapid changes faced in the environment. The womb, where a baby spends 9 months is a closed dark environment. The only sound is the soft rhythmic whoosh of the mother's heart beat.

At birth, the baby is suddenly exposed to the outside world with temperature changes, sounds and stimulation by other humans. Tired, fed up, frustrated, unable to speak and with limited motor responses, the baby responds by crying. Once started, like a stuck car horn, the wailing does not stop till exhaustion sets in. Colic eventually disappears spontaneously by the age of 2–3 months. It leaves the parents with distant unpleasant memories, which like labour pains are soon forgotten.

Sometimes crying may be due to a correctable cause like hunger, tiredness or a sudden noise which may have startled the baby. The temperature may be too hot or too cold. Clothing may be inappropriate for the weather. Diaper pins may be uncomfortable or they may be nappy rash. Babies are also sensitive to emotional upsets and conflicts in the house. Babies like body contact and cuddling and some may require more body contact than others.

Holding the baby as long as it is required provides the baby with a warm, secure, nurturing environment. It does not inculcate bad habits.

A baby weeping continuously should also be medically evaluated for some other cause of incessant crying, like an earache, intestinal or urinary problems.

If everything is normal, before reaching out for that OTC mixture, there are several harmless age old techniques that can be tried for soothing a fretful child

- ➢ Gently massage a little baby oil on the abdomen. Move the fingers clockwise around the umbilicus
- ➢ Swaddle the baby if it is cold. Alternatively remove the clothes if it is hot
- ➢ Give the baby a warm bath.
- ➢ Carry the baby on your shoulder crooning, singing or making rhythmic whooshing sounds near the ear
- ➢ Play soft music
- ➢ Reducing milk, caffeine and some vegetables (cabbage and cauliflower) in the mother's diet, though unproven, may help
- ➢ Emotional support for the mother is important as she may be mentally and physically exhausted, frustrated inadequate and unable to cope.

The WHO has recommended that babies be exclusively breast fed for 4–6months. This means that they receive nothing else, not even water.

Before administering "miracle" medications to normal healthy babies, for symptomatic relief of colic, please check the fine print for the alcohol content of the medication you are about to administer.

Chapter 45

Child Abuse _ It's Closer Home Than You Think

Sexual abuse makes headlines, but it is not the only form of abuse. There are other forms of physical abuse, when a stronger individual or group torments a weaker section. Abuse can occur obviously in times of war, and surreptiously in times of peace. Women, children and the elderly are always the worst affected and form the most vulnerable segments in society.

Many senior citizens do not have social security, an adequate pension or medical insurance. This leaves them financially and emotionally dependent on their children. Some are grateful for the care and nurturing they received in childhood. Others forget and not only fail to provide for their parents, they try to cheat them out of whatever they have.

Sometimes elders are denied adequate balanced nutrition. Their bodies show signs of malnutrition, anaemia, vitamin and mineral deficiency. They may not be helped with personal hygiene. If bathing becomes a problem they are left dirty. They may have to wear unwashed clothing. Physical manhandling may leave signs of bruising, cause head trauma or produce fractures in the brittle bones of the elderly. Constant ill-treatment may produce confusion and hasten dementia.

Women are physically weaker than men, and this has led to assaults and sexual violence against them. In many societies physical abuse within the marriage is condoned and sometimes respected. This leads to injury, chronic diseases and psychiatric ill health. In India, lack of education, awareness, government and family support has also lead to the widespread murder of young married women.

Sexual abuse of children occurs among both boys and girls. Contrary to popular belief, the ratio of abuse in both sexes is almost equal. In Mumbai, Delhi and Kolkata 6 out of the10 18–20 year olds surveyed had been sexually abused. Abuse is said to occur if there is inappropriate touching of any area of the body (not necessarily the genital areas) in a way that makes the child uncomfortable. Sometimes there is forced sex or masturbation. Physical injury or spread of STD (sexually transmitted diseases) may occur. The contact may occur repeatedly over a period of time.

Sexual abusers are seldom strangers. It usually involves a member of the family, a close friend, a teacher, a person working in the school or an authority figure. This leads to a psychological feeling of betrayal and abandonment. Appeals for help from other adults may be ignored or the child may not be believed. Fear of social stigma may lead to suppression of the crime. Also, in India, legal solutions are difficult, time-consuming and cumbersome.

Children may also be abused physically. They may be beaten with kitchen implements or sticks, threatened with knives, burnt with hot oil, or pushed into fires. Witnesses may be reluctant to get involved as it is difficult to distinguish between discipline and abuse, especially if the involved adult is the parent or the legal guardian of the child. Much of the abuse is accepted as "deserved" and is socially acceptable. Also, the definition of abuse varies in regions and countries. Exact statistics are difficult to come by as much of the abuse is covert and hidden. The victims in India do not have a 911 number to telephone. They have limited or no access to protection by the government or social organisations.

Also the abused children may be the biological offspring, step-children, adopted, or illegally employed domestic or factory labour.

Psychological abuse is more subtle. It involves constant nagging, "putting down" and comparison with more successful peers. It creates loss of confidence and a feeling of worthlessness. Sometimes it involves intentional confusion of gender identity, with a girl being dressed in boy's clothes and vice versa. It may involve derogatory remarks about skin colour or physical attractiveness.

Abused children are sleep deprived, have short attention spans, inconsolable crying and poor academic performance. They may have unexplained bruising or bleeding from the genital areas. Eventually they become violent insecure adults, unable to form lasting meaningful relationships. Some get addicted to drugs and alcohol. They seldom become productive or useful members of society. Many turn into abusers themselves leading to a vicious cycle. They are in need of psychiatric help, which is either unavailable or unaccepted.

As responsible parents we should not:

➤ Abandon our children and refuse to nurture them, even if it means sacrificing a busy social life.

➤ Employ children under the age of 14 years in factories, workshops, hotels or for domestic work. They are not physically capable of withstanding the rigors of long working hours. Mentally, children are immature and irresponsible.

➤ They cannot really be faulted for making mistakes or failing to follow instructions. Underage workers are not being provided charity, they are being exploited and their lives ruined.

➤ Paying for the education of such children in a charitable residential facility is more helpful and socially responsible.

We are the educated elite, the cream of Indian society. In the absence of any structured forum for tackling abuse, we have to listen to our children, speak up and act. We can prevent the physical, psychological and mental destruction of our children, who are tomorrow's citizens, and protect our senior citizens, whose past contributions have made our country what it is today.

CHAPTER 46

AMBITIOUS PARENTS

"Tinker, tailor, soldier, sailor,

Rich man, poor man, beggar man, thief.

There is a wealth of opportunity in today's world, with many jobs, callings and professions. Yet most often we hear, "This is my daughter, we are going to make her a doctor." Or, "This is my son; we are going to make him a software engineer."

Common words, praise worthy ambitions!

Yet you rarely hear "my son wants to be an anthropologist?" Or, "my daughter wants to do social work?"

Another set of parents abruptly terminate their children's education at the middle or high school level. Their excuse is "I do not want my daughter to travel by public transport. It is dangerous and the high school is far away. I have enough money. She doesn't really need a higher education."

Translated it means "I have already found a good match. How much education is after all needed to cook and run a house? With the same investment I can get her settled". Or, "my son needs to relieve me in the shop (or factory). He does not really need an education. After all, we have a profitable family business. He just needs to learn the ropes to be able to run it properly!"

Continuing an adolescents' education does not necessarily mean making them "pundits" in that particular field. Education is essential to acquire the social skills required to cope with life in the real world. Education teaches tolerance and involves interaction with individuals who are different culturally and socially, and come from diverse religious backgrounds. Education terminated before completing high school may permanently halt mental maturity at the same level.

Physical maturity is measured medically using a "Tanner" scale awarding points for the appearance of secondary sex characteristics like breast development, auxiliary and pubic hair and the appearance of the external genitalia. It does not necessarily correlate with either the chronological or the mental age of a teenager. An adolescent who looks like an adult physically often mentally lacks the coping skills required for independent existence.

The amount of guidance required at this crucial phase in life therefore varies tremendously. In addition, hormonal imbalances, mental immaturity or peer pressure predisposes teenagers to mood swings and irrational behaviour.

Teenage students are financially dependent, as, at the high school level, they attend coaching classes and tuitions paid for by parents, and do not have part time jobs. They are unable to think beyond the next set of exams. Their physical health suffers, as in an effort to "beat the competition", they have no time for games, leisure, hobbies or development of their individual personalities.

Teenagers have no independent financial resources to follow "their life ambition." Once parents have decided on a particular course of action, interests and talents are relegated to the back seat, as children have no option but to bow to adult pressure, meekly follow parental guidelines, and maintain family prestige.

Many of the teenagers lack the interest and motivation to follow the career path chosen by parents. Frankly, they are interested in something else, a career option, which in the parent's perception does not seem capable of eventually providing a financially lucrative future for the child.

Success, or "getting admission" on "merit "requires tremendous motivation and hard work. These two perquisites will not be present in a child uninterested in the parentally planned future and actually wishing to do something else.

Inadequate performance and failure is greeted by consternation on the part of the parents. Unable to face "failure" of their own ambitions, they "purchase" a seat for the unmotivated uninterested teenager in the parentally desired subject.

In this scenario, the financial implications and a feeling of lack of self worth emotionally burdens an adolescent, who though dejected and demoralized is unable to say, "I told you so."

The university or course may not be up to par, or in the desired geographic area, adding to the stress level.

There is the additional psychological trauma of having to cope with leaving the secure home with strict parental control and ready-made decisions. This unresolved tension leads to anxiety attacks, depression, mental breakdowns, and unimaginable stress levels. In some cases, suicide appears to be an attractive and viable option. Bewildered parents are unable to offer any solace or mental support.

A student, who did not make the merit list, is either not motivated enough or lacks the mental make up for that particular course or profession. Coercion to study and succeed only results in more failure. Rebellion occurs and is manifest by either a total failure to pursue academics, recourse to recreational drugs and alcohol or promiscuity.

All of the above are self-destructive.

Individual God given talents should be nurtured and utilized. All talents are not necessarily academic. Everyone cannot be professionals, doctors, engineers, dentists and architects. There are a host of other professions and options. Career guidance books are available in bookstores and information is available on the Internet.

Try to stress 45 minutes of aerobic activity for physical and mental well being. Regular exercise increases mental and physical stamina and confers an inner resilience. A physically active teenager who participates in sports as well develops a "team spirit," is motivated, competitive, can interact with peers and is better equipped mentally to deal with the roller coaster of life.

Parenthood does not automatically confer infinite wisdom, ability to judge or an ability to foresee the future.

Before you loose or child forever, listen!

We parents may be wrong. Try to see their point of view. Teenagers do have ideas hopes and ambitions. Sometimes they actually may be right!

CHAPTER 47

PARENTING IN A CHANGING WORLD

Anxious parents look and sound like clones, as they stand around saying "my child has just finished school; and is writing the all India competitive entrance examinations; to become a doctor, lawyer, engineer, dentist, architect, etc." For some of the parents and students this is the first time. For others, it is a stress producing second attempt after a year in an intensive coaching facility.

More and more parents are thrusting financially lucrative career choices on their children. Parents do this out of love, as they prefer to have their children trod a familiar path career wise, rather than have them sail in unchartered waters. They feel rightly or wrongly that they know what is best for their child. Often the career choice is based on their own frustrations, thwarted careers, unachieved or achieved success, or the desire to emulate an idol.

Sometimes intelligent children fail to qualify, as their own unmentioned career choice was different. They then lack the interest, inclination and motivation to complete the chosen course. Capitation fees used to purchase a seat for children who did not qualify on merit, places them under a tremendous amount of stress and guilt. If there is also academic underperformance, depression and parental pressure can lead to alcoholism, the use of recreational drugs, promiscuity, or suicide.

Wherever your child is going, and whatever course they have decided to join, there are certain checklists for the parents to follow, to avoid unneeded stress in both parties.

Check the fee structure and ensure that dues are paid on time. This avoids needless tension. It is the primary responsibility of the parent to support the child financially. Colleges may withhold hall tickets, or harass and humiliate students whose arrears are not cleared in time.

Drugs, drinks and sex are a great danger in college life. However, college students need some spending money to maintain friendships and develop personality. "Going Dutch" and sharing expenses equally is a good way to resist peer pressure. Having a reasonable amount of money keeps temptation at bay and reduces obligations in a world where there is no free ride. There are many shady ways to enhance income, temptations are plenty and opportunities abound.

A vehicle may be required for transportation. Make sure the child has a valid driving licence. If the vehicle is a motorized two wheeler, invest in an ISI certified crash helmet. A plastic eye guard, a cloth cap to avoid sunlight, a plastic rain coat hood, a jacket, or a construction helmet will not protect the head. It can crack like an egg shell if it comes into contact with a hard surface. This can result in death. Taking a friend pillion is common. It is difficult to refuse a "lift" o a friend class mate or colleague. The pillion rider should also be provided with a helmet. In the case of an accident, if the pillion rider is injured seriously or fatally, the child is left with a lifelong psychological scar.

Speak to the children and tell them drinking, drugs and driving do not mix.

Children see, hear and observe the actions and value systems of their parents. A smoking or alcoholic parent cannot really convince their children that these are not desirable habits.

A cell phone is now a lifeline. It can act as a security blanket. It helps if the child is stranded, in danger, in an unavoidable unpleasant situation, or ill. A basic cell phone with a limited fixed monthly bill is all that is required.

Food and vegetables provided in the mess may be over cooked and unpalatable. Try to make sure that at least two raw tomatoes and a banana are consumed every day in addition to the canteen or mess food. Try to drink milk as well. The government supply (Aavin) now provides disposable tetra packs which can be stored without refridgeration. If this is not available iron, B complex and calcium supplementation may be required.

Immunizations must be up to date. Adjustment during the first year of college is difficult enough without preventable infectious illness causing lack of attendance, missed practical classes and other problems.

> 16 yrs dt (diphtheria –tetanus) booster,
> 3 doses of Hepatitis B,
> 2doses of Hepatitis A,
> MMR (measles mumps German measles),
> Typhoid (booster every 3 years)
> Chicken pox vaccine (for those who have not yet had chicken pox)

These should all be given. Since there is a minimum one month interval between doses, the schedule should be started and completed well in time.

Mosquitoes are a menace and cause diseases like malaria, filaria and dengue fever. A plastic mosquito net should be provided. Long term use of mosquito mats, coils and mosquito repellents in a poorly ventilated room causes sniffing, sneezing, wheezing and other respiratory allergies.

Underclothes and socks should be washed personally daily in a bucket and not handed over to dhobis. This prevents "dhobis itch" especially in the groin area. It is an embarrassing irresistible urge to scratch caused by a combination of detergent and chemical allergy and superimposed fungal infection.

From the beginning of time, the emotions and actions "love" arouses have bee beyond rational comprehension. This is particularly true in the case of teenagers. Shouting, chastising, ridiculing, and forbidding are all self destructive actions. Support your child without criticism or encouragement. This is a difficult middle path to follow. Without the need to prove a point, or admit a self humiliating mistake, in the long run, this tactic may pay off as the "undesirable other" may then vanish of their own accord!

Support your children financially and emotionally. Write, e-mail or telephone daily, or at least three times week. This way, you will be "a concerned parent" conscious not only of the child's friends, whereabouts, progress and academic performance, but also their thoughts, feelings and moods.

Stay in touch! It will pay off in the long run!

CHAPTER 48

MEMORY BOOSTING IN CHILDREN

The father held up a white plastic bottle, shook it vigorously, rattled the capsules inside, and said, "The advertisement on television said that if I give my son one of these a day, his memory will improve. His marks are low. He studies hard, but cannot recollect his portions at all. In the mornings he cannot remember what he learnt the night before. Will this work?"

I doubt it.

Faith can move mountains, but in this case it was the parent who had the conviction and not the boy.

What exactly does contribute to good academic performance in school?

The answer is a good memory, analytical and mathematical skills, a secure productive home environment, and concerned interested and participating parents.

The human memory is like a computer, with temporary folders and permanent files. Facts seen and heard (auditory and visual inputs) are stored for a few seconds in a temporary folder, encoded, processed, and then retained in appropriate areas of the brain for later use and recall. It is an active and selective process during which unessential material is filtered out and discarded.

Storage is a biochemical phenomenon at the junction of the brain cells, mediated by enzymes like acetylcholine and glutamine. Reduction can occur in the manufacture of the enzymes. Sometimes, the encoding, storage, retrieval of facts, or some combination of these may be faulty. This may as a consequence of a disease like Alzheimer's, or occur as part of the normal aging process. In either case the memory deteriorates.

Memory loss or "forgetting" tends to occur if the material is not meaningful, interesting or arranged in a proper logical sequence. A string of incomprehensible nonsense is more difficult to remember than facts that are rational.

Trying to educate a child in a foreign language, or suddenly switching the medium of instruction from one language to another is therefore self-defeating. The child has to understand in order to retain. What he hears should not sound like meaningless cacophony if it is to be retained in his brain.

A positive attitude goes a long way to improving memory. Any educational presentations should be stimulating to the existing brain synapses. The child should want to make an effort to remember. To do that, there must be an interest in what is being taught and intent to remember a fact.

Understanding of new material depends to a great extent on awareness and how much is already known about the subject. It is easier to build up on existing knowledge than to learn something totally new. This is where the foundations of education must be strong with an emphasis on understanding the basics rather than rote learning. A fact can be remembered better if the logic behind it is emphasized and explained.

Just like the computer hard disc, our memories have a limited capacity. Valuable available space should not be cluttered with irrelevant insignificant data. Instead, the total amount and form of the material memorized must be selected based on importance of the portions. Learning and remembering improves if new knowledge and ideas are sorted into meaningful categories or groups (the correct folder).

Reciting data out loud both in the words of the book or in your own words, makes the auditory and visual synapses function in tandem (double input) rendering the memory more efficient. With constant use, a pathway becomes smooth and familiar. In the brain too existing neural connections can be beneficially strengthened by repetition.

Children can be taught mental visualization. It is an old yogic practice and a powerful memory tool. A mental picture (photographic image) of facts uses parts of the brain, (triple input) entirely different from that used by reading or listening.

Word and knowledge association also increases memory, when one fact is built on another and progresses in a logical sequence.

New facts produce new electrical and biochemical connections in the brain. These needs time to "set" and "gel" after it has soaked in. A review of the day's lessons in the morning before going to school helps this as it cements and reinforces existing knowledge.

Fatigue sets in at the enzyme level after a certain period of use. Time is needed by the brain cells to rejuvenate itself. A series of shorter study sessions, with timed breaks, distributed over several days is therefore preferable to fewer, longer, time intensive study sessions.

Constant television viewing, especially of cartoons, mindless soap operas and serials unnecessarily saturate the synapses responsible for short-term memory. Essential information, instructions and lessons taught in school cannot find space for storage and are rapidly "forgotten." Analytical skills can improve with solving puzzles, word association and memory games.

Mathematical skills improve with memorizing the multiplication table up to sixteen, and regular problem solving from the text book, as an extra activity, even when there is no math homework. Reading books, both fact and fiction, opens up and stimulates new areas in the brain (new folders).

Continuous tuitions for several hours a day, lack of regular physical exercise and daily recreation in front of the television are therefore counter productive. (The more they learn, the more they forget).

Structured aerobic physical activity for at least 20 minutes a day replenishes the micro enzymes in all age groups.

Memory training with proper techniques and a supportive lifestyle is the cure. It is not treatment with packaged herbal medicines or tonics.

"All work and no play makes Jack a dull boy!"

Chapter 49

"Watch Me! I Can Communicate!"

Babies are able to speak words that express their needs coherently (not gurgling) when they are about 15 months old, even though they speak their first word around the age of one. Until then, parents have to try to figure out what is wrong from the screams, facial expressions, crying or laughter. This is often very frustrating for parents, although some mothers read their children's body language better than others. This system totally breaks down when the infant is placed with a care giver, to whom the nuances of its body language make no sense whatsoever. No one is able to accurately answer the questions, "What is wrong? Are you in pain? What do you need? Are you hungry?"

After researching these developments, we spent a great deal of time and effort trying to teach our grandson to sign. He was not interested, and then realization dawned. We still live with domestic help, and often have relatives as substitute care givers. Most often every expressed or unexpressed wish of the child is fulfilled immediately. They do not need to sign!

Native American Indian tribes like the Cheyenne overcame this problem. Their speech itself was simple, guttural and rudimentary. Yet, they had a number of basic hand signs with which they communicated with each other from infancy to old age silently over long distances. In Native Americans, even though their language skills developed relatively late, their communication skills appeared before they could crawl. This was their way of adapting to a hostile and dangerous environment. Their survival was a question mark, and depended on rapid silent communication, comprehension and response to danger.

Necessity is the mother of invention. Recently, observation of the children of hearing impaired parents revealed some startling facts. Infants have a strong survival instinct, and in a totally hearing impaired environment, where loud screams evoke no response they adapt to signing very fast. The infants picked up sign language around the age of 8 months and were able to communicate adequately with their deaf parents. This is 7 months more before appropriate verbal communication is established.

Watching these developments, child care providers discovered that most infants can learn to sign their requirements as early as 5–6 months even if their parents can hear. They are able to use their arms and hands to sign.

Their motor skills developed far ahead of their verbal skills. They involve a totally different area of the brain. Also a single movement like putting the hand on the front of the chest can be taught to indicate hunger. It involves large muscles and does not require much co-ordination. The word "food" on the other hand involves complex movements of the small complex muscles of the tongue, soft palate and cheeks.

Emotional development starts at around the same time. Using colour computer scans to visualize minute blood flow changes in the brain researchers have now established that babies feel anger, jealousy fear and happiness. They respond to the environment. They have an ability to resolve "jumbled" pictures and are able to identify family members who bear even a slight resemblance to their parents or care takers. Infants lose this ability as they grow older. If they are able to sign, they are able to express their emotions adequately. This leaves them with less frustration.

An increasing number of parents are investing in educational CDs, DVDs and books to learn sign language and teach their children. These parents find that the toddlers observe and understand a great deal more about their environment than previously thought. If they can sign for a pleasant experience like feeding, and then they get what they signed for, the rewards for the parent and the child who have learnt to communicate and bond with each other are immeasurable.

Each family can evolve its own set of signs. Sign language can also be learnt from books. In teaching children to sign universal deaf sign language does not have to be learnt. Signs can be individualized for the baby and family. Most children learn a sign after it is repeated 5–6 times. If they are praised and rewarded for accurate signing they learn even faster. Soon they will learn to indicate "dog," 'toy" "food" "milk" "sleepy" or "wet diapers."

Signing provides an emotional bond in families, as siblings are often accurately able to express their needs and feelings to their parents and each other.

Signing does not slow normal speech. Children who learn to sign speak normally just like other babies. Parents who used sign language with their babies do tend to enunciate words more clearly when speaking to them so when they do start to speak the speech may be clearer. The emotional bond between signing children and parents is stronger. This is partly because these involved parents take the time to teach their children to sign.

Signing children spoke more clearly, were better disciplined, read more and eventually had a 10–12 point IQ edge over their peers. That eventually will make a great deal of difference in today's competitive world.

Signing can involve the whole family. This means everyone will able to communicate with the new baby. This reduces sibling jealousy. Nurturing and caring are less frustrating as the infant no longer has to resort to headache arousing screeching and screaming till the adults around can comprehend.

Never mind babies, silence is golden. Sign language may reduce the nerve wracking cacophony in our homes and work environment, reducing stress and increasing productivity.

CHAPTER 50

SCHOOL AND EDUCATION

It is that time of year again. Stressed out parents are standing in serpentine queues in front of books, shoe and cloth shops as they attempt to cope financially, emotionally and physically with the dawn of another school year. The transition from "cartoon network" holidays to "tuition filled" school days is traumatic. Adequate and timely preparation reduces the stress levels in parents and children.

The interests of child need to be safeguarded with an elementary checklist for parents. There is usually a whole month before school starts, so:

Get the immunization card verified by qualified medical personnel. Even the most meticulous parent gets caught out with incomplete immunization in these days of "package "immunization deals and "master" health check ups. The schedule has become complex with combined shots, varying intervals and boosters extending upto the 16 th year.

Many of the ailments acquired in school like jaundice typhoid, chicken pox, measles, German measles and mumps are preventable with timely and adequate immunization. This reduces the number of "lost" school days. With the large portions that need to be covered during the course of an academic year, missed days means that the child soon starts to lag behind.

Organize comprehensive teeth, eye and ear checkups. Visual defects and hearing impediments are not conducive to academic excellence. It may be a simple blocked ear as a result of wax build up or something more sinister. Poor eyesight uncorrected with the proper prescription glasses, with may result in difficulty in alphabets, numbers and copying from the board.

Establish a routine from the beginning. Wake the child up at 5 am and encourage 20 minutes of aerobic physical activity. Running up and down on the road in front of the house is safe and free. This will wake up all "sleepy heads", ensuring that they are "alive and kicking" for the rest of the school day. It also sharpens the intellect, improves memory, boosts academic performance, instils discipline and reduces stress. Unfortunately many schools do not have structured compulsory PT or games periods, especially in the higher "exam going classes." Games periods, already scheduled only twice a week, though theoretically present in the time table are usurped for 'annual day "practice or in order to complete the academic portions. It is therefore mandatory that the parent takes an interest and ensures sufficient exercise.

Homework should be completed the evening before. Portions taught should be revised again in the morning.

Remember children need around eight hours of sleep to remain healthy. Lack of sleep reduces concentration and marks.

Check the load your child carries. Books should be carried in a backpack with padded straps that fit well on both shoulders. The weight should not be more that 10 % of the total weight of the child. If it is more, the centre of gravity is altered. Balancing while climbing on and off a vehicle is difficult, precarious and can be life threatening. Some schools have opted for a "file system" reducing the notebook load. They allow textbooks to be kept at home, and arrange subjects so that only a few need to be taken to school each day. These recommendations can be brought up at PTA (parent teacher association) meetings.

Ensure that the child eats a balanced and hearty breakfast. This often is all that carries them through the day. Milk (200ml) should be given after breakfast and not as a substitute for it. If the child refuses t eat, then 1 oz (30 gms) of ragi should be cooked, milk and sugar added and it should be given as a substitute.

If there is a 10 AM break, a nutritious and preferably home cooked snack should be eaten. Indian cuisine has a wide variety of snacks like carrot halwa, peanut barfi, kesari, bhajis, samosas and bondas. Simple carbohydrate overloaded "instant" snacks like cream biscuits and crunchy salted preservative laden packaged eats should be avoided.

Many children attend "tuition" and "tutorials" straight after school. A banana along with another snack should be eaten as soon as school is over and before the grind starts. It is not possible for a tired hungry child to concentrate other wise.

Adequate drinking water should be provided from home. A child needs approximately 1.5 litres for a school day.

All the school uniform requirements should be purchased and tailored in advance. Children are penalized and suffer corporal punishment for a failure on the part of the parent to do this in time. Materials made out of 60%: cotton and 40 % polyester wear well and are suitable for our climatic conditions, especially as in many classrooms there is a single fan for 60 or more students. Undergarments and socks should preferably be made of pure cotton and washed daily. Sweaty socks "air dried" and worn again are a potent source of fungal infections of the feet. Shoes should be of good quality. Damaged torn worn out ill-fitting shoes damage growing feet irreparably.

Transportation to and from school should be safe and stable.. Packing 20 or more children into an auto rickshaw is not a pleasant, safe or advisable way to commute.

Television viewing should be restricted to two to two and a half hours on Saturdays (one movie). Watching 2–3 hours daily is a common cause of academic underachievement.

Have realistic expectations for your child. All children are different, with talents and interests that are individualized. There is no point in trying to fit all children (even siblings) into the same common mould. Failure to perceive this causes stress and depression in parents and children. Before berating and blaming a child for academic underachievement reflect, introspect and consider if the problem occurred because of your unreasonable expectations.

Attend all parents teacher meeting regularly. The regular physical presence of concerned parents prevents bullying, ragging, victimization and favouritism. Volunteer to help with annual days, plays and sports days. Teachers will remember your actions and your child will benefit.

With a little time and effort school days can be remembered as "fun days" and not fear and tension filled "bamboo stick" days!

CHAPTER 51

THUMB SUCKING

The ultrasound images were captured on film and beamed all over the world. It showed pictures of an unborn baby still in the uterus sucking vigorously at his tiny thumb. The image was cute; the photographs were published in many newspapers, readers looked, smiled and read on. Yet the very same adults make loud disparaging remarks when they see toddlers sucking their fingers. They make futile attempts to humiliate the child, and offer unsolicited advice to the cringing long-suffering helpless parents. Some pounce on the hapless child and yank the offending digit out of its mouth.

The search for food is one of the most primitive reflexes for survival. Sucking satisfies hunger. Some babies discover the pleasures of thumb sucking before birth and are actually born with calloused hands. After birth, almost 75 % of the children under the age of one suck their thumbs. In developing countries, with longer and more prevalent breast-feeding and late weaning, the incidence is less. Exact statistics are not known with certainty.

Thumb sucking occurs as it is a normal primitive pleasurable survival reflex involving the oral cavity, one of the most sensitive areas of the human body. It gives the child a warm encompassing feeling of security, self-sufficiency and independence. Thumb-sucking children are usually less dependent on their mothers and other caretakers. They are also emotionally secure children, contrary to popular opinion. Children in orphanages hardly ever suck their fingers.

Yet, for some unfathomable reason, thumb sucking is viewed a as "no-no" all over the world. Strangers pull the fingers out, scold, humiliate, or chastise the child. This is self-defeating, as in a single encounter, it is impossible to correct a primitive ingrained reflex. Parents obviously struggle with the habit. There is no need to advice them. No parent says "suck your thumb. Carry on! "

Thumb sucking is not a disease. It is harmless to society. Self-righteous adults also have oral fixations. They substitute cigarettes, alcohol or food for the thumb. These self-indulgent addictions are harmful to self, family and society.

Most children spontaneously give up thumb sucking by the age of two. Many continue, but exact statistics are difficult to obtain. The children are aware that this activity is socially unacceptable. They realize they are objects of ridicule among adults and peers. Hence thumb sucking becomes a subversive secret activity more enjoyable as it is forbidden. The habit becomes deeply entrenched. Thumb suckers usually eventually stop because their social lives become busy, with school and other activities. They no longer have the time or the privacy to continue the habit in secret.

Almost 50% of the original thumb suckers (75% girls) continue up to the age of 7 years and beyond. Giving it is up becomes more difficult, as constant sucking releases endorphin, which affects the brain, producing a calming euphoria. It becomes an addiction difficult to overcome and it satisfies unmet psychological needs.

Thumb sucking persisting after teeth start to appear causes the upper jaw to become deformed. A gap forms in the front and an "open bite" or "cross bite" develops, with crooked teeth and malocclusions. The nose is tilted upwards. Speech is eventually affected as the child begins to lisp, or speak indistinctly. Swallowing is inefficient and nutrition is affected.

The severity of the problem depends on frequency, intensity, duration and also the position in which fingers or the thumb is placed in the mouth.

Prevention of prolonged thumb sucking is not achieved by scolding, beating or humiliation. This only drives the activity into secrecy. Application of chilli powder or neem extract seldom works as the child soon learns to spit on the thumb and wipe it, successfully removing the noxious chemical. Socks or mittens do not work as the child soon learns to remove it.

Dentists can fabricate a plate to be placed in the mouth. This theoretically reduces the pleasurable sensation making the child give up the habit. It is expensive and usually does not work.

A painstaking effort should be made before the child goes to school. This prevents discovery by peers and subsequent humiliation. Success is a slow painstaking process. The child should want to give up the habit. Talk to the child and try to emphasize that a partnership with the parent will meet with quicker success. Try to tackle daytime sucking first.

- ➤ Give them a structured stress free day.
- ➤ Full fill the psychological and physical needs of the child with love and support.
- ➤ Respond and correct hunger, crying, tiredness and boredom. Meet their unexpressed needs.
- ➤ Distract the child without mentioning the habit as the thumb heads towards the mouth.
- ➤ Offer rewards for thumb free days.

Night time sucking is more difficult to tackle, as it may be a prerequisite for sleep. Try to remove the thumb after the child is in deep slumber. Covering the sleeping child's thumb with a band-aid may help.

Once the thumb sucking habit is broken it usually disappears for good. Rarely is it replaced by another bad habit.

Success is ensured with your love support and encouragement.

Chapter 52

Bed Wetting

Parents and care givers anticipate that their nocturnal diaper changing activities will be over by the time their children are two or three years old. They dispense with rubber sheets diapers and plastic underwear. Unexpected wet beds cause sleep deprivation, stress and frustration. Often all the children and the parents sleep in the same bed, and a deluge of urine in the night disturbs everyone's sleep!

Many parents invest a great deal of time and effort into inculcating toilet training and encouraging "dry" nights. They painstakingly make the children pass urine before sleeping. Some set alarm clocks and wake them up once more during the night. They keep hoping that "today will be the last wet day." Continuing "nocturnal enuresis" or "bedwetting" fills both the parent and the child with a sense of failure and shame.

Bed-wetting is said to be primary when bladder control has never been achieved and secondary when there is a reversion to bedwetting after six dry months. As the child grows older bedwetting becomes a social problem. Wet beds in hotels or in the houses of friends and relatives are difficult to explain and make travel embarrassing. Bedwetters become objects of ridicule among family members and peers if their failures are publicized. Sometimes families do this intentionally in an effort to shame the child into remaining dry at night. They feel that the bed wetting is intentional. Nothing could be further from the truth. Older children often do not wish to discuss their problem, and out of embarrassment, are not willing to seek medical help.

Urine collects steadily in a muscular bag called the urinary bladder. Once filled, the bag contracts and urine is forced out. In infants this occurs regularly during the day and night. It is an uncontrolled automatic activity. As the child grows older a hormone called anti diuretic hormone (ADH) is secreted at night. This slows the nocturnal urine production so that there is no over filling of the bladder. Urination occurs frequently during the day, infrequently at night and eventually stops altogether. Also, as the brain matures and develops, urination ceases to be spontaneous, and comes under higher control. Urination ceases to be indiscriminate and people are able to hold their urine till conditions are conducive to emptying the bladder. Some adults (especially men) feel that the whole world is a public urinal, and continue to perform indiscriminately on walls, trees and around the countryside.

Most children achieve night time bladder control by the age of 3, but around 30 % continue to wet their beds after that. Even without treatment this percentage falls to 20 % by the age of 6. However,1 % of adolescents continue wet their beds. Bed-wetting may be familial and is commoner in boys. In 80% of the cases there is a positive family history with parents and siblings having wet their beds through adolescence and sometimes well into adult life. These families accept the problem and wait for the children to grow out of it.

Some treatable conditions like urinary tract infection, diabetes, sickle cell disease and constipation predispose to bedwetting. It may sometimes be associated with the hyperactivity attention deficit syndrome. In these cases of secondary bedwetting tackling the primary problem cures the disease.

Daytime incontinence is commoner in girls and women. It is a different condition, with dribbling and soiling of underclothes occurring during the day. It occurs when the bladder is full, or if the abdominal pressure is suddenly increased with laughing, coughing or even talking. It occurs after child birth when there may be trauma to the urethra or damage to the nerve plexuses around the bladder neck. It is increased with obesity.

It is due anatomic differences between the male and the female. Males have two sphincters in the urethra so that better control is achieved. The female urethra is shorter and has a single sphincter.

In women with day time stress incontinence, bladder control exercises can help. The bladder should not be allowed to overfill. A concentrated effort should be made to urinate on time by the clock. The time between successive voiding can be gradually increased till accidents cease to occur.

The pelvic floor can be strengthened by doing Kegel's exercises. Squat on your haunches, lean forward, place the arms over the head so that the abdomen is pressed. Consciously tighten the muscles required to stop urination in mid stream. Each time, while urinating, stop and start several times in the bathroom, so that the sphincters become tight.

Wear panty liners if afraid that an accident may occur in a public place. They are smaller, compact, more comfortable and less expensive than sanitary pads.

Sometimes loss of ladder control and involuntary voiding may suddenly occur. This may be due a structural abnormality. It can also occur if the bladder capacity is less than normal either congenitally or as a result of repeated urinary tract infections. Tuberculosis can cause a small "thimble" bladder. This has a compromised reduced capacity and cannot hold much urine.

Sudden loss of control can occur because a child is too engrossed in an interesting activity to pay attention to distracting signals from the bladder.

If urine and blood test results are normal, and there is no structural abnormality, then the outlook for bedwetters is good. 15 % get spontaneously cured every year till puberty.

Berating the child, punishment or humiliation is not the answer to the problem.

A few simple measures also help.

➤ Limit the fluid after 7 pm. Do not enforce this too rigorously as then you will have a thirsty child who still wets the bed.

➤ Avoid caffeinated drinks (colas tea and coffee.) These cause an increase in urine output and spasms of the bladder muscle.

➤ Allergy, especially to chocolate and artificial colouring may cause a similar problem.

- ➢ Increase roughage (fruits and vegetables) in the diet to prevent constipation.
- ➢ Encourage the child to go to the bathroom before bedtime. If possible take the child to the bathroom before the parent goes to bed.
- ➢ Avoid punishment.
- ➢ Encourage success.
- ➢ Leave a light on in the bathroom, and en route, so the fears of the unknown do not prevent an essential visit to the toilet.
- ➢ Wear simple underclothes without complicated bows and zippers so that they can be easily pulled up or down quickly if required.

Bed wetters are usually sound sleepers. Their deep sleep ensures that nothing disturbs them not even the sensation of a full bladder. They tend to stay dry when staying overnight in unfamiliar surroundings. This may be due to the sleep being less sound because of anxiety. This fact can be used to motivate the child before sleeping by making then say "I will not wet my bed " loudly three times before sleeping

Nocturnal enuresis may suddenly reappear in a child who has been dry for more than 6 months. This may be due to a urinary tract infection, or the sudden onset of juvenile diabetes. Sometimes precipitating event may be difficult to identify as it is emotional. There may be anxiety and mental turmoil due to death of a parent, a new sibling, illness or a separation. There may be alcoholism, violence and physical abuse occurring in the family.

Medications can be used to treat bedwetting. They are successful. There is a tendency to relapse once the medical treatment is discontinued. Medications include nasal sprays and tablets of anti diuretic hormone, and antidepressants like imipramine.

Parental help support and perseverance ensures that most children attain bladder control within a year.

In any treatment regimen for this complex problem the most important ingredient is love.

CHAPTER 53

MEDICAL PALMISTRY

"Read your palm?"

Our bodies are unique, each one similar yet distinctive and different. Our eyes reveal character and are the windows of the soul, and our hands provide irrefutable evidence of our identity. Palm prints and fingerprints with characteristic whorls, arches and loops are unique, individualized and never identical in two people, even if they are twins. One of the oldest biometric methods of establishing positive identity is by using fingerprints.

Magicians and soothsayers understood that the lines on the palms, the shape of the hands, and the length of the fingers were distinctive. Palmistry soon became a profession as profitable as astrology.

Well-read, astute and experienced palmists can make shrewd observations of demeanour and body language. They accurately assess your mental health, character, physical capabilities, and life span. An obese unhealthy person is obviously not going to live long. An unkempt appearance reveals mental trauma. An agitated person or one with a drooping mouth is obviously depressed. People who consult palmists professionally usually have unresolved anxiety.

The medical fraternity has now accepted what palmists had been saying for centuries. A detailed examination of the palms does provide valuable clues to the medical history, lifestyle, diseases and life expectancy.

Palmar creases form during the 12 th week in utero, as the unborn baby holds its hands tightly clenched in the uterus. Normally there are three palmar creases or lines. Any physical, medical or drug-induced injury to the foetus at that time (first three months) is reflected permanently in these creases. Abnormal palmar creases formed by the clenched fist of the foetus can be clearly seen on the open palm of infants after birth.

Sometimes the upper two lines fuse to form a single palmar crease called the "simian line" which stretches across the open palm of the infant. It is associated with certain chromosomal anomalies. Of these, Down's syndrome, (trisomy21) or mongolism is the most common. Trisomy means 3, and in these individuals the chromosomal abnormality involves fusions and deletions on chromosome 21. There are other trisomies involving chromosomes 13 and 8 and in these too the palmar creases are abnormal.

Palmar creases can be picked up on ultrasound examination after the 12th week. If it is found, the foetus should be closely monitored for appearance of associated abnormalities in the kidney, heart or other organs.

A single palmar crease can be present in 1 out of 30 apparently normal individuals. It is commoner in males, and is usually present only on one hand, with the other palm showing normal creases. One or both parents of these children may have the abnormal crease on one hand. This is a minor aberration and warrants close monitoring. These children may reveal mild abnormalities in other organs in later life. There is also a 50% greater chance of developing leukaemia or some other blood cancer.

Marfans syndrome is a genetic disease in which the person has arachnodactly or abnormally long fingers like that of a spider. This can be diagnosed before birth by ultrasonographically measuring the length of the mid finger and hand.

Congenital hypothyroidism, certain renal diseases and some forms of dwarfism are associated with a tripartiate hand, with the index, middle and ring fingers being the same length.

People prone to chronic disease like leprosy and tuberculosis also tend to have only two lines on the palm, but their single abnormal line is just above the thumb.

People with mental illnesses have more open loops and less whorls on their finger tips.

Not all abnormal palmar creases are hereditary or genetic. Alcoholic women who continue to imbibe during pregnancy can produce children with "foetal alcohol syndrome," and a single palmar crease.

Cigarette smokers, and others suffering from chronic respiratory ailments, or those with congenital heart disease have discoloured nails, which may be blue. Some lung diseases like bronchiectasis, and chronic intestinal diseases and cause clubbing, and the nail acquires a convex parrot beak appearance. This disappears and the nail becomes normal when the disease is cured.

Jaundice causes the skin of the palms to turn yellow. Carotenemia, a harmless condition, caused by an excess consumption of yellow carotene containing fruits and vegetables, produces a similar appearance.

Hormone levels in the uterus influence finger lengths. A person (irrespective of the sex) with the index finger shorter than the ring finger will have had more testosterone (male hormone) while in the womb, and a person with an index finger longer than the ring finger will have had more oestrogen (female hormone). The difference in the lengths can as little as 2 or 3 %, but is nevertheless important. Professional women and female scientists tend to have higher levels of testosterone relative to their oestrogen level, making their brains closer to those of men in general. The converse is true with men working in fine arts and social sciences.

The position in which we hold our palms is a reflection of the BMI (body mass index). A BMI (weight in kg divided by height in meter squared) more than 30 is diagnostic of obesity. These adults tend to hold their hands with the thumbs facing backwards as they stand. Overweight people with a BMI between 25 and 30 hold their arms with the thumb facing sideways. People of normal weight with a BMI 20 –25 stand with the palms facing forwards.

With practice and attention to detail, you too can become an expert palmist!

CHAPTER 54

THE SHAPE OF EARS

Ears, Small Large Elephantine

Terrorists and other unsocial elements are caught even though they have radically altered their physical facial characteristics. They undergo plastic surgery, change their hair colour, grow moustaches and shave beards. Even then, they are recognized irrefutably before their fingerprints are taken. This is because although cosmetic surgery can drastically alter physical characteristics, they do not change the shape of their ears. Ears, like finger and palm prints, and dental records, provide an irrefutable biometric method of identification. With computer aided tools, identification now is even more positive.

This is the rational for identification photographs requesting the subject to present three-quarters of their face to the camera. Police photographs also ask for full face and profile.

Faces change as age advances. Eyelids sag, double chins appear, skin folds and wrinkles increase. Our ears composed of firm cartilage defy age, do not change in shape, but continue to grow through out life instead. This is why some wizened senior citizens appear to have disproportionately large ears.

Our brain has a mental picture of our outer ear or pinna. These function as ear trumpets protruding from the head on either side of the body. They collect sounds which are eventually meaningfully interpreted. Alteration in the shape of the pinna confuses the hearing centre in the brain. Hearing functions below par until the brain reorients itself.

Ears are formed in utero from a series of cell "folds" which fuse together in a complicated predestined sequence to give ears their shape and unique individuality.. Sometimes fusion does not occur fully, and a tiny aperture is visible in the front of the ear called a pre auricular sinus. This can remain throughout life without causing any discomfort. In some, it gets blocked with water, soap, dust and other debris. It then becomes secondarily infected, painful swollen and red, and requires surgery and antibiotics.

Improper fusion can leave small mobile skin tags in the front of the ear. They are not manifestations of "good luck" and require cosmetic surgery.

In India ear lobes are pierced, sometimes for both sexes, at an early age. It is often a social function and may be accompanied by tonsuring. The ceremony may have a religious significance, and conducted in places of worship or by pujaris.

The instruments used for both procedures are may not be clean or sterile and the experienced elder not medically qualified. The gold needle heated used traditionally for the piercing may or may not be fully sterilized. It may have been used for many years on generations of children.

Children are susceptible to tetanus and hepatitis B. Piercing should therefore preferably be done only after immunization with the three doses of triple antigen and hepatitis B have been completed.

The ear lobe is very soft and the needle goes through easily. A restless child may move suddenly so that the two ear lobes are unfortunately asymmetrically pierced. The position should therefore be clearly marked with indelible ink prior to piercing after the ear is wiped with spirit or the antiseptic povidone iodine.

There are several advantages to early piercing. The young child is less likely to develop keloids (unsightly hyper pigmented protrusions) at the site of the piercing. Once there is a tendency for the skin to form keloids, all successive pokes will be affected.

Adolescents and older individuals pierce the cartilage of their ears in several places and have numerous earrings in each ear. The piecing unfortunately is performed by friends, relatives and unqualified enthusiasts, often using a sewing needle and thread. This often causes infection of the cartilage of the ear. If untreated it form a bag of pus. The entire ear can then be destroyed forming an unsightly "cauliflower ear" identical to the ones seen in injured boxers.

The ear and the kidney develop at the same time (around the 12th week) in utero. An insult in the form of an illness, prescribed medication or recreational drugs in the mother can affect both at the same time. The ear, unlike the kidney, can be clearly seen. If the ear is abnormal the kidney should be evaluated. The hearing should also be checked.

In normal ears, a straight line drawn from the outer edge of the eye should pass through the upper 1/3 of the ear. Low set are seen in Down's syndrome (Mongolism) and some other congenital conditions. Ears may be also be rotated abnormally, asymmetrically located and have extra creases and folds. Protruding (elephant ears) are normal, run in families, and can be corrected by plastic surgery.

A crease sometimes appears in both ear lobes. Called the "ear lobe sign" in medical parlance, it is associated with elevated lipids and cholesterol. Both ears turn black as age advances in persons with alkaptinuria or homocystinuria. In uncontrolled gout, "tophi" get deposited on the earlobes and are diagnostic markers for the disease.

Look closely at ears; you might pick up what your doctor missed!

CHAPTER 55

DIET AND EXERCISE — HOW MUCH IS ENOUGH?

The commonest mistake—underestimating intake and overestimating expenditure.

Do you suffer from diabetes, hypertension, have high cholesterol and lipids? Or is your BMI (wt in kg/ height in meters square) greater than 25? In short do you need to loose weight? Do you have to control your blood sugars? Or, do you just want to stay fit?

Age catches up with all of us. Even if you are young and fit and the ideal weight now, remember that your body is in a dynamic equilibrium with food intake (calories consumed) and calories expended.

The balance tends to tilt upwards as age advances, due to a marginal increase in intake over expenditure. This occurs inadvertently as the body metabolism slows down. Also, distances walked and stairs climbed decrease with professional success. We tend to use elevators and motorized transport. House work becomes less physically taxing with affordable appliances and domestic help. Eventually the weight creeps upwards in a never ending spiral.

Just take a look at the Life Insurance charts. For the same height, the normal average weight is higher for an older person!

Interested? You have probably taken the first tentative step to better health and a better tomorrow.

The point is – Do you know how?

Diets and miracle gadgets advertised on the internet, in magazines and on television offering magic ingredients or miracle diets to reduce weight or contour certain parts of the anatomy. Sea weed wraps, steam baths, "natural" adhesive patches and vibrating belts all seem safe and effortless.

Do these work? Is the expense worth it?

It is not practically possible to sustain heating habits different from that of the rest of the family. Once the diet returns to normal any weight loss benefit disappears. There may actually be a re-bound weight gain instead!

Also some diets are positively harmful. They upset the body's natural equilibrium and lead to dangerous conditions like ketosis. People sue the propagandists of these diets regularly abroad, but our consumer courts are not that progressive as yet.

Remember weight loss is actually based on pure mathematics.

Food eaten (calories consumed) minus exercise (calories expended) determines the eventual weight gain or loss. To loose weight you need to eat 20 calories/kg/day, to maintain your present weight 30 calories/ kg day and to increase your weight you need 40 calories/kg/day. Pregnant and breast feeding women needs to take 30 – 35 calories/kg/day.

This calculation has to be reset as you loose weight. For example, 20 calories/ kg is 1400 calories for a 70 kg adult trying to loose weight. As the weight falls to 65kg the requirement falls to 1300 calories a day. A reduction of 3500 calories results in the loss of ½ kg. Around 6500–7000 extra calories are needed to increase weight by 1 kilo.

Does that sound like a great deal of food?

➢ One idly is 85 calories and it equals 2 phulkas, ½ dosai, 1 slice of bread,½ cup of cooked rice, ½ cup cornflakes, ½ cup uppmav, ¾ cup of cooked vegetables (no oil), ¾ cup vegetable salad, 1 fruit, ¾ cup of cut water melon, 150 ml of skimmed milk, 1 square of chocolate, 20 peanuts, 20 potato chips, ¼ cup of chocolate ice cream or a ¼ " square of chocolate cake.

➢ Each teaspoon of sugar adds 20 calories.

➢ Oil, irrespective of whether it is sunflower, corn oil, soya, rice bran, groundnut, sesame varies only in the PUFA (polyunsaturated fatty acid content) and EFA (essential fatty acid) content, and adds invisibly but tastefully to the calories in cooked food at the rate of 45 calories per 1 teaspoon (5 ml).

Put simply, in addition to your normal diet, 2 extra squares of chocolate a day (2 chappatis) will eventually result in the gain of 1 kilo in a month, and 12 kilos in a year!

It is easier to mentally count calories if you work on the principle of equivalents. Once you are clear about equivalents and substitutions, you can probably figure out a palatable way to loose weight.

Natural foods like fruits and salads are complex, require digestion and increase the blood sugar levels slowly increasing the feeling of satiety. Simple sugars like honey, jaggery, sugar and glucose need practically no digestion at all, satiety is less, leading to greater consumption and hence weight gain.

Think of this before you reach for the bottle of fizzy flavoured sweetened calorie loaded bottled cola . It contains 100 calories for every 200 ml consumed, and all of it is in the easily digestible readily assimilated simple form!

A sustainable weight reducing diet is one which provides about 1200 calories per day. A diet containing 800 calories a day may ensure initial rapid weight loss but cannot be sustained on a long term basis.

Around 400 calories / day can be worked off with exercise and this results in a weight loss of 1 kg in around 2 weeks (24 kg /year) if a 20 cals/ kg/ day diet is maintained at the same time.

It is probably best to calculate the amount of time that you can spare and then utilize it maximally and efficiently. Vigorous exercise, (sweating and an inability to speak except in short bursts) pedalling on a stationery bicycle, using a rowing machine or treadmill works off around 10–12 calories / min. Walking consumes 5–7 calories/ min as opposed to running fast 11 calories / min, rapid stair climbing 14 calories/ min, swimming 8 cals/min, yoga, stretching exercises and low impact aerobics, 6 cals/min. Most house work utilizes 6 calories/ min and watching television or attending meetings a miserable1 calorie / min!

Calories can be worked off in exercise, but exercise alone without diet restriction will not result in significant weight loss. Conversely, diet alone without exercise will eventually result in weight loss, but neither will you be healthy nor look robust. Both will result in initial weight loss and then a tapering off of the benefits. The body adapts to this artificial famine, and then the weight starts to increase again.

Summer, with long days and vacations is a good time to embark on a changed alternative healthy life style with more outdoor physical activity, and less snacks and sedentary television viewing, even if it is the cricket test match season!

CHAPTER 56

AGE HEALTH AND ACTIVITY

"Puthro Rakshathi nardakye" (Children take care of the aged)

The lady's face was puffy, her feet oedematous, and she bulged out of her tight fitting blouse. Her husband looked no better, as he lurched in on arthritic knees with drooping shoulders and a down turned mouth. Her blood sugars had spiralled out of control and his blood pressure was high. As a couple they had managed to keep their illnesses under fairly good control until about a year ago. They used to walk in briskly together smiling at everyone else in the waiting room.

What has set off this chain of events? Could it be depression?

"Are your children all right?"

"Oh yes, our son has a good job in Canada. He sends us more than enough money every month. We can now afford domestic help, watch television and relax. As a matter of fact, he insists we rest, lie down and not do any physical work at all".

Good intentions, disastrous results!

The Indian population has crossed the 1.1 billion mark, and 7% are over the age of 60. People now live longer, have access to health care, enjoy better nutrition and education. Our life expectancy is steadily increasing. The retirement age however has remained unchanged and people stop working even though they are healthy and have plenty of productive years left.

At the same time, unfortunately, we do not have structured efficient social security or health care systems. Family members, in the productive age group (15–60), often have to shoulder the burden of caring for the over 60s. Often out of misplaced affection, filial duty and ignorance they insist that their parents "lie down" all day to "rest, relax and recover" from a lifetime of hard work.

Senior citizens must remain active to stay healthy. Each hour of walking adds a day to your healthy life span. Activity reduces risk of heart disease and cancer, helps control of diabetes, and reduces high blood pressure. Body weight remains under control. Bones, muscles, and joints stay flexile reducing the pain of arthritis. Physically active people have better coping skills and are less likely to succumb to anxiety and depression. Life becomes pleasurable. This in turn reduces the number of visits to doctors, medications and hospitalizations. Activity requires motivation.

We lack safe traffic free roads, parks and jogging tracks. Walking on a busy street with poor eyesight or hearing is not safe or advisable. It is better to find a quiet well-known road not too far from home. Measure a circuit and then calculate the number of times it has to be traversed to make up the required recommended distance. The average adult step is approximately 45 cms.

The ideal distance is 4 km, and it should be to be covered in 45 minutes.

If you find it impossible to leave the house, spot walking is equally effective. Mark a figure of 8 with chalk on the floor and walk on it alternating the directions clockwise and anti clockwise.

Jogging is pleasurable, efficient and there are very few contraindications to slow jogging. Start by walking 15 steps and jogging 5 steps for 5 minutes. Gradually increase the steps jogged, and the time taken, at two-week intervals until the entire distance (4km) is covered in 45 minutes.

Invest in a good sturdy pair of walking shoes and athletic cotton socks. This is a worthwhile investment as it will prevent injuries to the feet and the heels.

Muscle strength should simultaneously be built up. The arms and legs of the elderly have fat and bone covered with skin and no intervening muscle mass. Strengthened muscles hold joints in place and prevent misalignment and arthritic pain. Muscles efficiently utilize glucose. Rest reduces muscles mass, so that less glucose (energy) is used. The same amount of food then pushes the blood glucose levels higher in diabetics, necessitating an increase in medication or insulin injections.

Spend a few minutes doing muscle-building exercises. A "baby dumbbell "weighing one kilo is sufficient and available in sports shops. If you cannot find it, use 1./2 kilo packages of rice or dhal in a bag. They work as effectively and are available pre-packaged in shops.. Do the exercises like a school drill holding the dumbbells. Initially attempt 10 repetitions and gradually increase to 20.

Muscles should be stretched before and after activity. Stretching movements are demonstrated in the exercise programs on the television and can also be downloaded from the Internet.

Injuries should not be a problem if early warning signs like pain or giddiness are taken seriously. If important telephone calls may be missed while you walk, invest in a cell phone and take it with you. Boredom can be relieved by listening to music or religious discourses available on CD and cassette. These portable gadgets are not a prerogative of the young!

Some days will inadvertently be missed. Once three consecutive days have been missed any acquired benefit would have been lost and a new beginning has to be made. Maintaining health should be a priority. As time marches on, we just have to try harder, to go faster, and longer; to achieve the same goals and maintain what we have.

Too little exercise with too many excuses is the straight broad and quick road to ill-health and misery.

We all belong to God's army. So keep your body fighting fit.

Chapter 57

Osteoporosis

Short stooped and bent double

Some of our senior citizens are stooped and bent, while others appear shorter than they used to be. This appearance occurs in both sexes but is commoner in women.

It is due to weak and brittle bones caused by a preventable condition called osteoporosis. Initially, the onset of osteoporosis can be missed as it is painless and asymptomatic. It becomes noticeable only when the back starts to hurt or there is a sudden fracture of the vertebrae, wrists, hips or other bones. The diagnosis can be confirmed by measurement of the bone density.

Bones are made of calcium obtained from the diet, mainly milk and other dairy products, fruits like the custard apples and green leafy vegetables. Before the carcinogenic effects of chewing paan were publicized, a great deal of the calcium Indians obtained was from the lime used on the betel leaf.

Calcium is deposited in the bones between the ages of 25 and 30 forming a bone bank. With increasing age and the onset of menopause this bone is gradually lost causing primary osteoporosis. The bones become brittle and porous. The spine collapses on itself making the person appear shorter. Slight trauma, like bending over and lifting a heavy object, a small contact injury or fall a can cause a fracture and disability. The commonest sites for fracture are the spine, hip and wrist.

Primary osteoporosis occurs in both men and women with increasing age. It is six times commoner in women. This is because after menopause as there is a decrease in the level of the circulating protective hormone oestrogen which helps to build bones.

The risk of developing osteoporosis is increased:

- ➤ In the older age group
- ➤ menopausal women
- ➤ If there is a family history of osteoporosis
- ➤ If the initial bone bank developed between the ages of 25–35 was insufficient.

The recommended calcium intake is between 800–1200 mg a day. Calcium supplements are available as tablets and should be taken as most Indian diets are deficient.

Secondary osteoporosis can occur as a side effect of medications like the corticosteroids. These are often prescribed for ailments like arthritis or asthma. Some patients are not aware that they have been given steroids on a long term basis. Sometimes it is part of the unlabelled medication dispensed by practitioners of alternative medicine. Patients may self-medicate over a long period of time as the initial therapeutic dose offered immense immediate relief.

Some antacids contain aluminium which acts as a "bone poison" and interferes with the incorporation of calcium into the bones.

Thyroid disorders or malfunctioning parathyroid glands increase the risk of developing osteoporosis.

Lactose (milk) intolerance is common in India. It may be relative, where small quantities of milk are tolerated but an increased intake causes pain, bloating and diarrhoea. This results in an inadequate intake of milk and dairy products with subsequent calcium deficiency.

Malabsorption disorders may prevent absorption of calcium from the intestines. Common disorders are several forms of colitis, chronic diarrhoeal diseases and parasitic infestation. Some renal diseases prevent efficient utilization of ingested calcium.

An efficient deterrent to the development of osteoporosis is regular consistent weight bearing aerobic exercises. Children and adolescents should be encouraged to be physically active. During adult life walking, jogging or running for 30 minutes a day six days a week is probably sufficient. Exercise strengthens muscle mass, which proportionately increases bone density. It also improves coordination and this reduces the risk of falling and developing fractures. Some exercises like weight lifting are inappropriate as they can cause minute painful fractures in osteoporotic bones. Swimming is good for general fitness but not for bone deposition.

Yoga or simple stretches should be done in addition to maintain balance and flexibility.

Body weight should be maintained in the ideal range. Obesity increases the risk of both arthritis and osteoporosis. The converse is also true. Excessive dieting and exercise can decrease bone mass. With a proper balance between diet and exercise, the bones, muscles and heart get a good though not excessive work out.

Exercise can be incorporated into the daily routine by walking short distances instead of using motorized transport. Periodic stretching throughout the day will help keep muscles limber and help prevent muscle fatigue and strain.

In women Hormone replacement therapy after menopause was initially very popular as it appeared to reverse many of the adverse health effects of menopause. It has side effects, and is now used only in selected women on a short term basis under strict medical supervision.

In men androgen replacement with testosterone is also gaining popularity. It builds muscle strength and bone mass.

There are new classes of selective oestrogen receptor modulators (SERMS) like raloxifene , and other drugs like calcitonin, bisphosphonates and parathyroid hormone which selectively act on the bones and can also be used. They and have less adverse side effects. They can be used in both men and women.

Instead of hormones natural supplements have gained popularity. Common ones are evening primrose oil, ginseng and natural soy products. They contain isoflavones which can be used by the body as oestrogen. Tropical wild yam also reverses menopausal symptoms like hot flushes. Studies have been undertaken but they are inconclusive. The advantages are anecdotal and as yet scientifically unproven. Action on the bone is debatable.

Osteoporosis has the same incidence as breast cancer. Unlike the latter, with a little effort it is totally preventable.

> ➢ Maintain an ideal body weight
> ➢ Exercise six days a week
> ➢ Take calcium supplements

Age gracefully, not stooped and bent, but standing ramrod straight.

CHAPTER 58

WALK FOR LIFE

Mankind walked its way to the top of the evolutionary pyramid, past other mammals and our closest relatives the great apes. We were able to hunt food over long distances, overtaking other primate relatives with less developed calf muscles.

Indians with their analytical brains, multi-linguistic capabilities, lateral thinking and capacity for innovation, are capable of scaling unimaginable heights in the global economic scenario. Yet, our evolution is going to come to stand still if we do not keep up our endurance training. We are developing diabetes, hypertension, and high lipids, and dying of "heart attacks" in the 20s and 30s. We do not reach the peak of our achievements. Nor do we fulfil our dreams and desires. Asked to exercise, we have a ready excuse, "I just do not have the time doctor, and you cannot imagine how busy my life is!"

Everyone's life is hectic, even that of people who sit in front of the television all day watching serials have a demanding scheduled life. They cannot bear to miss the next episode!

Starting to walk is easy; basically all that is required is will power and an end to procrastination.

- Walking first thing in the morning has many advantages.
- Later during the day other activities may prevent you from walking.
- Muscles resting all night need to get "kick started."
- Mental and physical performance for the entire day gets a kick start..

Start slowly for 10 minutes a day during the first week, on the road in front of your house. The area is safe and the surroundings familiar. The pace should be fast enough to make continuous speaking of a complete sentence difficult. Imagine that you are late for an important appointment and keep that pace. Develop a rocking rhythm, with no jerks. Pumping the arms increases the efficiency and the calories consumed.

Increase the rate, time and distance of the walk every week until you reach the target of 4 km a day in a time of 45 minutes. First concentrate on the time and then try to increase the speed. Doing double the distance on weekends and other holidays adds a boost to your heart and exercise schedule.

- ➢ Maintain a proper upright posture the head straight.
- ➢ Breathe through the nose with the mouth closed.
- ➢ Do not clench the hands into fists.
- ➢ Try to achieve 80% of the target heart rate. This is measured as (220 –age) X80/100. eg. If the age=30 220–30=190. 80% of 190 =152.

Injury can be prevented by stretching before and after exercise. Although this may seem like a waste of valuable time, but it definitely prevents damage to the muscle and increases their efficiency.

To warm up stand upright, interlock the fingers, and raise arms straight above the head. Stand on the toes with the knees straight. Next, flex the front leg at the knee, Extend the back leg. Alternate the legs. Hold each position for a count of 30. Repeat 5 times.

Walking does not require a fitness centre, with separate unsuitable inconvenient timings reserved for women. It is efficient as a solitary activity without friends or relatives. Talkative companions reduce walking efficiency and increase the time taken. Tardiness on the part of companions, lack of motivation and inconsistency increase stress and hence reduce effectiveness.

Investment in loosely fitting sweat absorbent cotton clothing allowing the legs freedom of movement is necessary. If perspiration is not allowed to evaporate, the body heats up. If the legs do not move freely the pace of walking gets reduced and entanglement in clothing may result in a fall.

The onset of diabetes or hypertension may be inevitable due to a genetic predisposition. It can however be delayed by 10–15 years with regular and judicious exercise. Asthmatics and those with air pollutants in the work place can increase their breathing capacity and reduce frequency of wheezing attacks with regular walking.

Daily exercise cultivates regular habits with the person wanting to sleep, wake and exercise at regular hours. This reduces fatigue, limits stress and increases endurance. The adrenaline and serotonin produced by the active calf muscles combats depression and accentuates brain activity. The morning metabolism gets kick started, providing a better boost than a caffeine laden cup of tea or coffee. This in turn contributes to success in academics and in the work place.

A person's life expectancy can be calculated based on genetics, family history, diseases present, life style and aerobic exercise activity.

Each year of exercise adds approximately a year of life if consistency is maintained. If exercise is discontinued any accrued benefit disappears in around 3 days. It then becomes increasingly difficult to restart a once successful schedule.

In senior citizens, and those leading a retired life it is very easy to lie down and relax. There are many pertinent excuses, lack of energy, traffic, time constraints, house work schedules. Eventually, lack of physical activity first makes it difficult to climb, then walk, then stand, or even sit for long periods. Ultimately, they spend long periods lying down producing muscle atrophy, postural (hypostatic) pneumonia, and eventual death.

Start walking today for a healthy tomorrow.

CHAPTER 59

OILY FACTS

Oil is essential for life. Cell membranes contain oil and it helps to keep the cell wall rigid, water proof and intact. It is also necessary for the absorption and transport of fat soluble vitamins. It is a constituent of bile which helps digestion. It acts as a replenishable source of energy.

Unfortunately we have developed a taste for the flavour which various oils impart to food. This prevents our body from regulating our intake. Consumption is based on greed not need. Attempts to keep the total cholesterol: less than 200. HDL cholesterol (the "good" kind): over 40, and LDL (the "bad" kind): less than 100 are then not successful.

All oils contain saturated and unsaturated fats, in addition to some essential fatty acids in various ratios and combinations. No one really agrees about the type or amount of oil that can be consumed for healthy living.

The Italians and the Greeks swear by olive oil. They are convinced that it is responsible for everything good in their lives, like their handsome looks, longevity and energy. Olive oil does reduce the level of LDL cholesterol; prevent arteriosclerosis, blockage of arteries, and high blood pressure. It also increases the secretion of bile and facilitates the absorption of the fat soluble vitamins A, D and E. Unfortunately it is prohibitively expensive in India.

Groundnut oil is almost as good as olive oil in providing a "heart healthy diet." Inadequately refined peanut oil is occasionally contaminated with non edible oils for higher profits by unscrupulous retailers. Also, ground nut oil has been implicated in mild and severe allergic reactions in some susceptible individuals.

The Bengalis feel that nothing can compare with the subtle pungency that mustard oil imparts to the cooking. The Tamilians argue that sesame oil is best. Both these oils have a low content of saturated fatty acids. Mustard oil contains a high percentage of erucic acid which may cause cardiac problems. Sesame oil does not have that problem, is popular locally and internationally, and is widely used in Chinese cuisine and as a salad dressing.

During all these arguments about various cooking media, the Malayalees maintain a discrete silence. They have to. They may (as they claim) eat the tastiest food in the world, but it is fried in coconut oil and laced with more fried shredded and sliced coconut. Coconut oil has a very high content of saturated fats and this pushes up the cholesterol and triglyceride levels of the user. Coupled with financial success and an inactive lifestyle, a high proportion of the population in Kerala have heart attacks and strokes in their twenties and thirties. Yet, this unhealthy oil makes the food so tasty that it does not seem a bad way to go. Some of them would rather "eat well and die young!"

Palm oil initially gained a great deal of popularity as it is cheap and has a composition is similar to that of coconut oil.. In addition it contains some protective antioxidants and retinoids.

Sunflower and the related safflower oil also are widely advertised and are popular as cooking media good for the heart. They have the highest percentage of "double bonds" in each molecule.

In Japan for many centuries a favourite cooking medium has been rice bran oil. It has a nutty flavour which enhances the taste of deep fried foods. It contains anti oxidants and vitamin E which prevent cancer. Awareness has increased about its hidden benefits and it is now being increasingly used in the fast and processed food industry.

A personal homemade oil mixture, incorporating all the good in each type of oil can be made

Mix 1 litre refined groundnut oil 1 litre sun flower or saffola,

250 ml sesame oil, 2

50 ml rice bran oil,

50 ml coconut oil

100 ml olive oil.

This can be mixed stored and used. Each member of the family requires around than 2 tsp of oil a day. A family of 4 therefore requires 40 ml of oil (5 ml = 1 tsp) a day or 1.2 litres of oil per month.

The human skin needs oil to keep it moist prevent flaking, scaling, cracks and secondary infection. Oil applied to the skin externally keeps it supple and makes the person appear fresh and glowing. In Japan women who constantly apply rice bran oil have an unwrinkled waxy complexion. In India as we are exposed to the tropical sun, we should protect our skin by applying oil.

A good mixture for the skin is 500 ml coconut oil, 500 ml sesame oil, 150 ml of rice bran oil, 100 ml of olive oil 100 ml of almond oil. Apply a small quantity, let it soak in for half an hour and wash off.

You too can become a shapely, ageless, unwrinkled, rice bran beauty with unclogged arteries.

Chapter 60

Sleep Deprivation

"Sleep is reversible death. Death is permanent sleep."

This thought must have been reverberating in the subconscious mind of the lorry driver as he dozed at the wheel, veered crazily and swerved abruptly into the path of the oncoming car. The car brakes screeched, but it was too late.

Two fatalities, one cause.

The driver probably had to reach his destination within a specified time. There was no substitute driver. There are no laws stating how much a driver should sleep before driving lorries or taxis. There are no laws regulating the rest timings professional drivers. Enforced insomnia leading to daytime fatigue and drowsiness, leads to sudden attacks of unavoidable slumber in the midst of activity. Even without actually dozing off, lack of sufficient sleep increases reaction time and prevents proper decision making leading to judgemental errors and accidents.

Everyone has an occasional inadvertent or intentional sleepless night. For most people, this is not a problem. In10% of the population, it becomes chronic with difficulty in falling asleep, remaining asleep through the night, or early wakening. They then become "just too tired," to function. This results in absenteeism, daytime drowsiness, inadequate performance, poor concentration and fewer promotions.

When the job involves driving or operating machinery, drowsiness and a slow reaction time is life threatening! In others, it may be just an embarrassment during work, gatherings and social functions.

Why does this occur?

It may be due to unregulated hours of work, or because of trouble falling asleep, or lack of restful sleep. The formerly is avoidable the latter two have to be tackled.

Sleep is not simply the absence of wakefulness. It is a complex state of active and coordinated brain processes the total amount and composition of which changes throughout life.

So how much sleep is enough?

The best measure of the amount of sleep needed is how you feel upon awakening. If you awaken feeling refreshed, it is enough for you. It shows an individual variation from 4 to up to 10 hours.

Infants and children normally sleep 16 to 20 hours a day, adults (till 60) sleep 7 to 8 hours a day and, after that, adults sleep approximately 6 hours a day.

The deepest and most refreshing kind of sleep diminishes with age, the lightest sleep, increases with age. As a result sleep in old age becomes more fragmented, with brief awakenings causing people over 60 to experience some degree of insomnia.

Constant daytime drowsiness or early-morning awakening is not a normal part of aging. The fact that older adults sleep less than younger adults may reflect their inability to sleep, not their sleep requirement.

Problems with sleep may be unavoidable, as in those who do shift work. This causes a disturbance in the normal "circadian" sleep-wake rhythm and chronic insomnia. To maintain a normal rhythm the person requires adequate exposure to natural or artificial bright lighting at the times that the body considers "day" and "night".

Medical conditions like hyperthyroidism, the restless leg syndrome, urinary tract infections, arthritis, peptic ulcer, bronchial asthma and hot flushes (in menopausal women) cause frequent awakening and relative insomnia even though the time spent in bed is more than adequate.

Alcohol, (either too much or an abrupt withdrawal), interferes with sleep. A "drink" at bedtime may induce sleep, but its narcotic effects are a misconception! The amount of REM (restful) sleep is inadequate after a drink, and there is early awakening. The sleep is not refreshing.

Nicotine (cigarettes, beedis, snuff, chewing tobacco), caffeine (cola drinks, chocolate) produce mild forms of exhilaration and are not conducive to the mental relaxation required for sleep.

Psychological problems like grief, anxiety worry, depression and unresolved stress prevent sleep.

Some medications cause insomnia as a side effect.

For "a good nights rest":

➤ Establish a regular bedtime in a quiet, dark, cool bedroom conducive to sleep, without appliances emitting electromagnetic waves like a TV or computer.

➤ Do not lie in bed out of boredom. If you cannot sleep get up and do something like reading or watching television.

➤ Regular exercise, especially aerobic, has been show to make people fall asleep faster and produce deeper and more restful sleep, but should not be done in the last two hours before going to bed as it then tends to produce paradoxical excitement.

➤ A light snack like warm milk or toast which contains the natural sleep inducer L-tryptophan is often helpful.

Circadian rhythm disturbances can be corrected through exposure to bright light for two hours at a time to shift the body's timing mechanism and produce onset of sleep at a "typical" bedtime. Get up at the same time every morning even if you have had a late or sleepless night, and eventually you will be sleepy at the right time. After a sufficient number of days, your inner clock will be sufficiently adjusted.

Some social problems causing stress and insomnia cannot be avoided but have to be confronted head on, and tackled either with yoga, meditation and prayer. If all this fails there is always a psychiatrist available.

Sleeping tablets should be taken only by prescription and that too as a last resort.

If you're having trouble falling asleep, wake frequently once you fall asleep, or wake up earlier than you want to, try using acupressure on one or both of these points. The spirit gate is below the little finger at the wrist and the inner gate is two and a half finger widths below the wrist at the centre. Maintain the pressure for one minute.

Happy sleeping!

CHAPTER 61

STRESS

A help or hindrance—the choice is yours!

"Everyone hates me and is against me! It is not my fault! I can't cope, or sleep, I'm too stressed out to function."

Familiar feelings?

Stop ! Don't reach out for that sugar, caffeine or nicotine fix! You are probably just suffering from unresolved stress like 70%of the population!

We all produce chemical messengers to our brain called serotonin, cortisol and noradrenaline. Maintaining a controlled correct balance between these chemicals keeps us stress free.

In a sleep deprived partying workaholic (16 or more hours of activity per day), there is no time for the body to automatically adjust the levels of these chemicals. This results in unresolved and continuous stress, a feeling of being "out of control" which produces elevations of the wrong chemical messengers to the brain, and negatively impacts health.

The rate at which this chemical balance is achieved and adjusted varies in families. In 10 % of the population it does not occur efficiently enough. They have inherited a "low stress tolerance" and cannot handle "normal everyday problems". They live in a permanent unhappy state of stress, "give up" on life, loose interest in their careers and fail to realize their own potential or benefit society.

Stress is precipitated by unanticipated change in daily life. The change may be imaginary (worries) or physical (illness and injury.) or due to a normal hormonal changes occurring during adolescence, pregnancy, menopause or andropause.

The present society itself is stressful, relying on "information" instead of "experienced elders "to provide solutions to the problems in life.

Stress can have physical manifestations producing "aches" in the head, stomach and back; weight gain; constipation or diarrhoea, no sleep or too much sleep, high blood pressure, palpitations, tiredness, mood swings, resentment and depression.

Properly handled stress has a positive side, producing new perspectives, motivation, forcing action and meeting deadlines. In short, whether stress is a help or hindrance depends on our reactions.

Coping with stress can be naturally achieved by allowing the body time to rejuvenate and to recycle the chemical messengers after each stressful event.

Unable or unwilling to do this, artificial stimulants are used to cope and "boost" up the body's level of the required chemicals.

Substances commonly misused are:

➤ Simple sugars like glucose, lactose (milk sugar), fructose (fruit sugar), and sucrose (cane sugar) which are easily and rapidly absorbed by the body. A sudden rise in blood sugar leads to an immediate elevation of mood.(The medical profession also subscribes to this and administers "glucose drips" for that "weak feeling").

➤ Caffeine, found in coffee, tea chocolate and colas.

➤ Alcohol increases aggression, energizes and induces sleep. Alcoholics may eventually take a drink to "fall asleep", another to "get going" in the morning, to feel more assertive, or to make social gatherings "more fun."

➤ Tobacco, marijuana, cocaine, amphetamines, and heroin are potent addictive chemicals that directly boost brain function. These chemicals act rapidly and produce high energy levels, a false sense of well-being, with a quick and efficient boost. Unfortunately there is a equally rapid rebound effect with lack of energy, fatigue, aches and pains. In addition, adaptation occurs to these substances, so that the quantities consumed have to be gradually increased, from one cup of coffee a day, to a pot, or from smoking two cigarettes a day, to a pack, or from one drink a day, to a bottle.

Subconsciously, stress makes people reach out for sugar rich foods like a slab of chocolate or a cup of hot milky sweet coffee unaware that an artificial "sugar high." This is followed by a "sugar low" as the blood sugar fluctuates widely. People who have "food and alcohol binges" eventually end up with wild mood swings and bizarre behaviour. They fluctuate between being pleasant, happy and energetic to moody, depressed and anxious. This paves the way to weight gain, and loss of self esteem.

Stress can be tackled by keeping the blood sugar level normal. An easy way to do this is to avoid the simple sugars and eat complex carbohydrates (cereals, rice, bread and potatoes) instead, as these require digestion and assimilation. If the helpings are also small and frequent, the sugar is released slowly over a longer period of time, keeping the blood levels stable and hence the stress level low.

To reduce stress:

➤ Make your life regular with as little change as possible.

➤ Give yourself a break at regular intervals.

➤ Reduce social engagements

➤ Regulate the number of working hours

➤ Keep your blood sugar steady

➤ Eat vegetables (vegetables contain L Tryptophan which in its natural form is a stress buster).

➤ Remove cigarettes and alcohol from the house.

➤ Exercise regularly, preferably, something that brings you into contact with other people, at least three times a week.

➤ Do stretching or yoga and meditation for at least for 20 minutes a day.

In today's world, in the course of a lifetime, a person has to be flexible enough to handle a tremendous amount of development, adjust to an environment dominated by change, achieve a stress free balance, sleep well, and be energetic, productive and joyful.

All this is possible with a little effort to modify an unhealthy lifestyle.

Good Luck!

CHAPTER 62

CONSANGUINITY

Dangerous Liaisons with Close Relatives

"My husband is my uncle, my grandmother my mother in law, my mother my sister in law, and my children my niece and nephew. Who am I?"

This is not a riddle!

It is a common identity problem caused by marrying a maternal uncle. Marrying the mother's youngest brother is an accepted social custom in South India. It is not considered incest, nor is such an alliance forbidden by society.

In some other areas, marriages are arranged between cousins, but not uncles. In other regions, alliances are forbidden from the father's side of the family as those genes are believed to be stronger!

Relationships between individuals become blurred and confused as a consequence of the inbreeding and consanguinity (a relationship between two people who share a common ancestor) prevalent in our society.

16% of the marriages in India are consanguineous. The incidence varies from 6% in the northern states to 56 % in Tamil Nadu. This high rate of consanguineous marriages is closely mirrored by birth defects and genetic disorders in the population. It is 40 times higher in Tamil Nadu than in any other state in India.

Under the Hindu marriage act passed in 1955 a legal marriage can occur only if the bride and groom are separated by five generations on the father's side and three on the mother's, unless local customs dictate other wise. This leaves a large loophole, legal prohibitions are meaningless, and uncles can, and are, still marrying their nieces!

Unrelated women who marry into a large family pose a threat to its unity. If a man's relationship with his wife becomes more important than his solidarity with his siblings, the couple might well take their share of the property and leave the larger group, thus weakening the strength of the lineage. This problem is solved with consanguinity. Any dowry, property or marriage settlement returns to the family coffers and the total wealth remains undiluted. The wife will not be an "outsider," thus reducing a man's likelihood of being pulled away from his family. She is less likely to be divorced by her husband, and more likely to be protected by her own extended kin.

Despite our fast paced moves towards modernity, networks of family are still the foundations of wealth, security, and personal happiness. Loyalty to family and caste cuts against the authority of the government or the advice of medical personnel. People see no reason to turn from this proven support base.

We can only hope that these customs will automatically decline with education and knowledge empowering women, marriage at an older age and smaller families. In this scenario, the eldest grand daughter will no longer be combatable age wise with the youngest uncle.

Human beings have about 35,000 paired genes in precise locations called "locii", one of each pair is inherited from each parent. The more closely two people are related, the more genes they share.

An imperfect or diseased gene is always weaker than its stronger counterpart. This means that the dominant (normal) gene will suppress the recessive (weaker) gene. Although the person carries the gene, they either do not manifest the disease or else it appears in a very mild form, often compatible with a normal life.

Genetic disorders in children occur when both parents (apparently normal) carry the same abnormal gene; both pass on the faulty gene, the child receives a double copy and exhibits the defect.

1st degree relatives: (parent/child; brother/sister) ½ of the genes are the same. 2nd degree relatives (uncle/niece) share ¼ of their genes. 3rd degree relatives: first cousins, 2nd cousins share 1/32 of their genes. As successive generations marry within the same family the number of shared genes becomes greater.

The most common form of a consanguineous marriage is between first cousins. The risk for a hereditary disorder for a child of such a couple is around 6 percent. This risk increases proportionately if the inbreeding has been prevalent for more than one generation.

If a child receives a faulty gene from both parents, then it results in a particular defect. If on the other hand they inherit one faulty and one normal gene then they become carriers without the disorder just like the parents.

Everyone carries faulty recessive genes, and we are all reservoirs for potential genetic disorders. These genes are innocuous in the heterozygous (mixed) state.

However, if paired with another faulty gene of the same type (homozygous state), they are capable of causing genetic diseases. The majority of serious genetic disorders are recessive, which means that an individual must inherit two copies of the abnormal gene (one from each parent) for the disorder to be expressed. Related parents are more likely to carry the same genes.

If sufficient defective genes are present (lethal combination) then people have a spectrum of problems, from increased rates of abortion, stillbirth and infant mortality. This makes it all the more important to submit still born children for autopsy despite sentimental feelings at the time. Any defects can be picked up and analysed. The results of such tests can be followed up to prevent recurrence and protect future progeny.

Sometimes, transmitted hereditary disorders may not be fatal. Defects like learning disabilities, impaired sight and hearing, an abnormal appearance, short stature, mental retardation, are combatable with a normal life span. They do however result in increased morbidity and medical expenses. Te affected child and parents find it difficult to cope in today's fast paced world. It takes its toll on the mental, physical and financial well being of the parents.

Common recessive diseases are beta thalassaemia, sickle cell anaemia, congenital adrenal hyperplasia, cystic fibrosis, phenylketonuria, i, alpha 1 trypsin deficiency. Some X linked (attached to a locus on the X chromosome) disorders are muscular dystrophy, haemophilia congenital adrenal hyperplasia. These are carried through the X on the mother's chromosome and exhibited in the sons. The sons show the disease the daughters carry it forward to the next generation.

Then there are the polygenic multifactoral hereditary disorders like schizophrenia, diabetes , hypertension, congenital heart disease, anencephaly, spina bifida meningomyelocoele, and other neural tube defects, deafness, blindness and some familial cancer syndromes. Cancers linked to genes have also been identified like breast and ovarian cancer, colon cancer associated with polyp formation and certain types of leukaemia. These genes are not precisely identified but the diseases obviously run in families.

Some diseases are mild and act only as irritants in the effected person's life, like a 6th finger or toe, abnormal ears, a misshapen head, cleft lip, learning disabilities and some kidney problems.

Irrespective of the cultural norms, we should do our part to ensure that we do not knowingly pass on faulty genes. Our children receive the best start in life that we can give them in today's competitive world.

Legislation alone will not succeed, and society has to voluntarily decrease the customs of marriage between close relatives generation after generation, with increased awareness of the potential hazards of such unions.

CHAPTER 63

THE TRUTH ABOUT SOYA

The soya industry has been advertising, publicizing and promoting the consumption of various products prepared from the soya bean. Propaganda states that soya milk is easily digested and that soya is a good source of protein, free from cholesterol and low in saturated fats. It also contains high concentrations of several anti-carcinogenic compounds the phytoestrogens and isoflavins.

Soy flour is added to bulk wheat flour and used to make chappatis. bread and biscuits. This is unwittingly consumed by the unsuspecting public. Soya protein is also promoted as an inexpensive meat substitute.

There is no disputing these relevant facts.

The Chinese discovered the benefits of the soya bean more than 4000 years ago. They consumed it like we do today, in several forms, such as tofu, chunks, mince flakes, miso, soya sauce, soya oil, and soya milk.

Soy protein is prepared by spinning or extrusion, dehydrated and then cut into small chunks or ground into granules. It can then be flavoured. Preparation for consumption involves mixing it with water and allowing it to stand for a few minutes. It can be used as such, or fried, or mixed with other vegetables. Milk is made by soaking soya beans in water and then straining it to remove fibres.

Traditional soya sauce is made by fermentation of the beans for a year. This destroys soy toxins. Commercially available soya sauce is very different. It is mass produced by the hydrolysing soya flour and then colouring it dark brown with caramel.

The lower incidence of breast and colon cancer in China and Japan has been attributed to the high consumption of soya products. These women also complain less about menopausal symptoms like hot flushes. Exactly how much is a cultural variation is not known or studied. Also many of these facts are actually misinterpreted. The Chinese and Japanese diets did not include large quantities of soya products as propagated. Soya was actually consumed by the poor Chinese during times of famine. At other times, small quantities of soya flakes or chunks (about a tablespoon) were added a few times a week to supplement and bulk the food. Weak soya milk diluted and consumed by the elderly in lieu of tea.

Also the soya products commercially available now, the tofu and soya sauce has very little resemblance to the traditional soy consumed in the east.

Today, vegetarians and health food faddists consume large quantities of soya protein believing that it is harmless, healthy and that it will reduce menopausal symptoms. Soya tonics and dietary supplements are aggressively marketed.

In adults, consumption of large amounts of soy products produces alterations in the hormonal balance in both men and women. This is due to the phytoestrogens in soy which are converted in the body to both oestrogen and anti oestrogen. The effect depends on the stage in life. Pregnant vegetarians, consuming large quantities of soy have higher incidence of genital tract birth defects in male children.

Soy contains isoflavones which stimulate oestrogen receptors in the breast. This can cause secretion of breast fluid, and stimulate abnormal potentially cancerous cells. Peri-menopausal and menopausal women with a family history of breast cancer or abnormal mammograms should probably avoid soy. By consuming an excess of soy products women are placing themselves at risk of contracting cancer instead of being protected from it.

Also no conclusive controlled studies have yet been dome to determine exactly what constitutes a safe intake of soy in adults.

Soy milk is available as a powder. It has to be reconstituted using three level scoops for 90 ml (3 oz) of boiled cooled water. No extra sugar should be added. Reconstituted ready to drink soya milk is also available in cartons and tetra packs in the supermarkets.

The soy propaganda has violated the WHO code and stated that soy formulas are superior to breast milk. It has also been advocated as a weaning food and easily digested "top up" supplement for inadequate breast milk.

The nutritive properties and long term effects of feeding soy formula unnecessarily to normal children is unknown. However it is known to contain agents which decrease thyroid function and predispose thyroid disease in later life. It also affects the sex hormones in boys and girls. No large long term studies have been done on how much of the extracts of soy can be consumed safely by children.

The Israeli government has issued a public health warning about the excessive unnecessary long term use of soy products especially in infants and children. Soy supplements are not longer OTC products in New Zealand. They have to be specifically prescribed.

Soy milk can be used for infants who are lactose intolerant and cannot tolerate breast milk, cow's milk or powdered infant formulas. Some children are genetically lactose intolerant. Others develop temporary reversible lactose intolerance, after an episode of viral or bacterial diarrhoea.

Think! Discretion and common sense are required before making diet alterations and lifestyle changes.

Watch out for opportunistic businessmen who manipulate facts to make a fast buck. Listen to your body before following new food fads. What it has to say is probably correct.

Chapter 64

Probiotics

Curds, Yogurt and the Probiotic Question.

The pharmaceutical representative was sure that the particular brand of antibiotic and the vitamin supplements he was marketing was superior to anything else in the market, "We" he said leaning forward persuasively, "as a company policy add probiotics to everything."

"Do your products cost more?"

"Yes, but think of the immeasurable benefits."

Probiotics are in the news, and are promoted as natural protective, anti-infection agents that boost the body's reserves against disease. In many countries they are widely advertised and sold on the internet and in pharmacies as capsules and powders that contain Lactobacillus bulgaricus and Streptococcus thermophilus. They are publicized as the good bacteria which promote health, versus and the bad bacteria that produce disease. Detailed instructions are provided on how they should be swallowed, usually with non-chlorinated spring water on an empty stomach.

Despite their fancy names and expensive packaging probiotics are not new products. They have been around for centuries.

The commonest probiotic is lactobacillus, found in curd or yogurt. This can be made at home by the traditional centuries old method of adding a "seed" (1/2 tsp) of live lactobacillus cultures (old curd) to warm milk and then allowing it to grow.

Commercially available yogurt or curd sometimes does not contain live lactobacillus as it may turn the product sour. The multiplication of the bacteria are controlled at a certain point by heat.

Probiotics like curd have many medicinal properties that are being rediscovered now.

After doing controlled studies, yogurt or curd was found to have an action in the mouth itself. By reducing the numbers of plaque forming bacteria , it reduces bad breath, tooth decay and troublesome, painful, recurrent, mouth ulcers.

In the stomach it helps to neutralize the gastric acidity, thereby reducing eructation, burning and dyspepsia. It prevents infection, growth and multiplication of the dreaded H. pylori bacterium. H. pylori is responsible for gastric ulcers and recently has been implicated in the eventual development of gastric malignancy. It also protects the mucosa and prevents development of atrophic gastritis. This prevents deficiency of vitamin B12 and development of anaemia.

In the intestine, it lives in symbiosis with other protective intestinal flora, reducing flatulence and also the incidence of diarrhoeal diseases. It is particularly useful in shortening the duration and symptoms of various viral diarrhoeas. It prevents constipation. It reduces the incidence of the irritable bowel syndrome. The immunological effects reduce the incidence and symptoms of Crohn's disease and ulcerative colitis. The transit time of food through the intestine is normalized. This makes bowel habits regular. All this helps in reducing the risk of colon malignancy.

The B –complex vitamins are synthesized in the intestine by the action of the probiotics on the digested food. This action provides the body with essential B-complex vitamins naturally and reduces vitamin deficiencies. The skin looks healthier, and ugly fissuring at the angles of the mouth do not appear.

Children need to be given breast milk for a year and to be exclusively breastfed for at least 120 days. Due to unforeseen circumstances, if artificial feeds with cow's milk or formula are introduced, the incidence of diarrhoeal diseases dramatically increases. In children who are given curd in addition to the formula, the incidence is less.

Many Indians are relatively lactose intolerant and develop bloating, abdominal pain and diarrhoea with ingestion of milk.

They tend to curtail their milk intake, and, in the absence of calcium supplementation, eventually develop osteoporosis as they get older. In curd, the milk is already partially digested, reducing the symptoms of intolerance. This facilitates intake. As little as 8 0z (1cup) of curd a day is beneficial in the prevention of osteoporosis.

There have been some studies which show that taking curd prevents the development of itchy vaginal fungal infection (candidiasis) in women. This can be precipitated by taking antibiotics. Other studies have shown conflicting results with no real benefit. This has not prevented pharmaceutical companies from advocating swallowing lacto bacillus capsules for candidial infection, or even more unpleasant, inserting lactobacillus pessaries in the vagina.

Curd also boosts the immune system. Regular eaters swear by it, saying the number of infections they suffer is less and the duration of illness is reduced.

The healthiest diet for the heart is the Mediterranean diet, with its unsaturated fat, high fibre and yogurt. This was what the traditional Indian diet was like, till we moved to a high fat low fibre fast food life style. Perhaps it is time to revert to eating curds and exercising 40 minutes a day to reverse some of the damage we have done to our metabolism.

Do we really need to purchase probiotics, or pay extra to have them surreptitiously added as spores to our prescription antibiotics and vitamins?

Apparently, 8 0z of curds a day is cheaper, more natural, and will do the trick just as well!

Chapter 65

Healthy Eating and Spices for Health

Studies have also shown that octogenarians (people over 80 years of age) consistently eat only 80–90 % of their total caloric requirements. None of the Guinness record holders for aging are overweight. In short, the quantity of food consumed affects total life span.

Recent studies have shown that obesity is bad for your health and career. Fat people, are less likely to be hired, more likely to be fired, less likely to be promoted and achieve lower targets than their normal sized peers.

Eating habits depend on availability of food, with too much causing obesity, and too little, starvation. Relative starvation can occur in the midst of plenty, in individuals with poor dietary habits, unscientific weight reduction diets or food faddism.

A change in weight of 1 kg, increase or decrease, requires an alteration in the consumption of 3500 calories. It is possible to eat nuts, sweets and other high calorie foods and increase this amount in the diet. Without caloric restriction it is impossible to "run, walk or work this off."

Too much of anything is bad. Carbohydrates and sugars produce obesity, diabetes and dental caries. A high fat diet, with excessive cooking oil or red meat, is associated with cancer of the breast, prostate and colon.

Food can be increased in bulk without much increase in the calories by eating food with a high content of fibre. A consumption of 30 gms a day is recommended. It can be achieved by consuming fruits vegetables and potatoes. Healthy dietary fibre consists of non-starch polysaccharide (NSP) which contains cellulose, hemi-cellulose, pectin and gum. These are undigested by dietary enzymes in the stomach and intestine. Fibre therefore produces a feeling of satiety, and prevents constipation by increasing the bulk of the stool. This in turn reduces the risk of colon cancer, lowers blood lipids and slows down sugar absorption. This is particularly beneficial in type 2 diabetes.

Healthy eating does not just mean reducing the quantity of fats or maintaining a correct caloric intake. It also means eating a balanced diet from all the food groups, with micronutrients, minerals and anti oxidants.

Yellow and orange fruits and vegetables (papaya, carrot) and greens like spinach contain anti oxidants and carotenoids. These protect against epithelial and colon cancer and heart disease. Antioxidants also delay chromosomal breaks responsible for aging.

Beneficial cooking additives are:

➤ Garlic which improves immune function.

➤ Curd restores normal intestinal flora after disease or antibiotic therapy.

➤ Lime contains vitamin C (ascorbic acid) which boosts immunity and stimulates liver function.

➤ Onions eaten raw or cooked contain antioxidants, restore normal gut flora and help in cold, cough and bronchitis.

➤ Coconut with its high content of saturated fatty acids promotes weight gain.

➤ Coconut water (not milk) is excellent for rehydration in diarrhoea and vomiting.

➤ Bananas provide calories as easily digestible complex carbohydrates and are beneficial in diarrhoea and mouth ulcers.

Herbs and spices not only add taste and flavour, but also provide us with many benefits. There has now been resurgence in their medicinal use. Small quantities added to the diet can complement and supplement medical treatments for acute and chronic diseases.

➢ Cinnamon and cloves help in mouth ulcers, toothache, nausea, vomiting and diarrhoea. A chewed clove keeps your mouth smelling fresh.

➢ Coriander and turmeric are antioxidants. They improve digestion and stimulate the appetite. Turmeric also acts as an intestinal antiseptic. It offers some protection against Alzheimer's. External application of some varieties of turmeric (Kasturi manjal) has a beneficial effect in certain types of acne.

➢ Ginger, dill and fenugreek relieve nausea, flatulence, and abdominal cramps. This in turn improves digestion and stimulates the appetite.

➢ Mint and curry leaves have antioxidant properties.

➢ Tender neem leaves, tulasi leaves and phyllantus niuri eaten daily are anecdotally protective against dengue and liver disease.

➢ Sometimes food contains carcinogens which are added intentionally. Lack of adequate government regulation makes some foodstuff dangerous.

➢ Harmful nitrates are used as preservatives, and are added to jams, squashes and commercially available pickles.

➢ Regular excessive consumption of ajinomoto is associated with stomach cancer.

➢ Substandard non-food grade carcinogenic red and yellow colouring matter is added to foods to enhance their visual appeal.

➢ Poorly stored food grows harmful fungi. Mouldy raw peanuts contain the liver carcinogenic aflotoxin.

➢ Cola drinks are contaminated with pesticides.

➢ Plastic water bottles and food containers, even when manufactured from food grade raw material deteriorate over time releasing carcinogenic dioxins. This can contaminate stored food and water and cause slow poisoning.

➢ Unregulated environmental pollution has now resulted in even breast milk, both human and cow, containing unacceptable levels of pesticides and harmful chemicals.

Recommendations for good nutrition are based on observations, studies and mathematical calculations, whereas dietary habits depend on culture and the availability of food. All over the world people are now becoming aware of the health hazards of some cuisines, and discovering that spices, herbs and some additives not only add to the taste but also provide health benefits.

Allopathic medicine has come a full circle. Doctors today are beginning to employ a holistic approach to disease. Successful treatment today requires integrating social, cultural, and dietary aspects of illness.

Some "old" remedies do work, and some traditional food habits are based on scientific facts.

CHAPTER 66

ALTERNATIVE THERAPY AND CHANGING CHOICES

Illnesses in people are the result of infections, genetics, environment or lifestyles. A person's response to disease depends on cultural and social influences and is influenced by the mental state of the person, with depression aggravating severity and duration of illness.

In this era of specialization, there are only a few family physicians, with the time and the knowledge to fit all the pieces of the diagnostic jigsaw together. Patients sometimes have to make a tentative sometimes erroneous diagnosis themselves with little expert guidance. They then gravitate to various specialists, spend a great deal of money and obtain little relief. This is particularly true if the symptom is an incidental manifestation of a disease process belonging to a totally different speciality.

The medical consultation itself may be expensive and exhausting, with an array of "essential" tests and uncomfortable procedures. Treatment may require swallowing nauseating multicoloured capsules and tablets. Relief may be incomplete, slow, and frustrating. The disease itself may be fatal, or incurable and require lifelong treatment. Treatment may involve adherence to discipline and behaviour modifications for the rest of the patient's natural life span.

Allopathic physicians are busy, and the skills required to communicate to non-medical persons are not taught in medical college. A tense, anxious and unhappy individual is often not willing to accept abrupt communications about chronic diseases at face value.

Brusque replies are common, with instructions like

"You have to take medicines for the rest of your life."

"This diet? It is forever!"

Sometimes, these answers are offered without any clarification, explanation or instruction. The physician's blunt answers and recommendations may be hard to stomach, especially when they involve radical changes in a pleasurable life style and include unpalatable dietary restrictions. The doctors themselves may be in a hurry, with other sick patients waiting, or it may be late in the day.

Snacking, smoking, drinking, chewing tobacco, taking paan enjoying gutka are not only forbidden, but held are held up as the root cause of all ailments. Sometimes, the disease itself, (as in the case of diabetes, hypertension, high cholesterol or cancer) is incurable. This may come as a shock to a person used in their younger days to time bound self- limited fevers, aches and pains.

Fortunately in India patients are presented with many alternatives in their quest for a cure.

There is the ancient "Aryuvedic Medicine" where herbs are administered to treat the patient. Much of this system of treatment is now documented and taught in colleges of alternative medicine. Traditionally treatment in this system was passed on to generations by word of mouth. The emphasis was on holistic healing, with diet, lifestyle changes, yoga and advice consistent with the cultural beliefs. A "guru –sishya" method of teaching was followed..

Many of these medicinal herbs are useful at a time when rational basis of therapy and scientific evaluation were unheard of. Unfortunately the exact method of action of these herbs, their metabolism, eventual elimination from the body, therapeutic doses and toxic levels has not been studied. Nor are there double blind placebo controlled scientific studies to evaluate their effects. When they are administered in the "natural form" the strength of the active chemical varies making titration difficult and dosing unpredictable. Some of the active chemicals in herbs like aspirin, digoxin and quinine are now extracted or chemically manufactured, purified and administered in accurate doses in allopathic medicine.

In the Sidha system of medicine the emphasis is on heavy metals like mercury, sulphur, copper, arsenic silver and gold and some herbs. Imbalance in the body's "vatham, pitham and Karpam" (metabolic cycles) are believed to produce disease. Balance is obtained by prolonged dosing with small quantities of metals.

Allopathic physicians used metals like arsenic and mercury to treat syphilis, gonorrhoea and other sexually transmitted diseases before the antibiotic era. These treatments fell into disrepute as it was found that the there was a very small margin of safety between toxic and beneficial doses. Elimination of heavy metals from the body is slow. They tend to get deposited in bones, hair, nails and internal organs like the liver kidney and bone marrow. Eventually toxic level and slow poisoning occur.

A change for the better or worse in the human body is slow. In both systems of medicine cures are not dramatic. Cures are anecdotal and not scientifically documented.

In today's world, neither the treating physician nor the patient has the patience to wait for a slow sustained and effective relief. Also, the herbal and metal preparations in both systems are manufactured in factories, and not made personally by the treating physician in back room pharmacies; as was the case in ancient India. There medicines are not under the purview of the drug controller. This leaves room for malpractice by unscrupulous traders as they randomly add allopathic medicines or steroids to the original formulation.

Training in each system of medicine is rigorous and specific. Just as an architect can design a building but only a rocket scientist can launch a satellite, each physician trained in a system of medicine should practice only what they have learnt.

Sometimes, despite these facts, alternative therapy seems to be an attractive advantageous option. Treatment is often culturally acceptable, highly recommended by friends and neighbours, with anecdotal evidence of "total" cures. Bottles of strange coloured liquids and little white tablets seem easier especially as diet exercise and blood tests are not required. Alternative treatment is symptomatic

– stomach pains irrespective of the cause, one liquid, menstrual irregularities another.

Unfortunately many of these treatments are unproven and unscientific. Herbal medications, (the little nameless white tablets and unlabelled mixtures) may have serious side effects that appear insidiously. Heavy metals used in some preparations may be slow poisons. There is no compulsion to take the treatment. There is no documentation of treatment medication or procedures by the patient or practitioner. The practitioner cannot really be questioned if side effects appear, as treatment was voluntary.

Alternative medications may be combined by the practitioner with allopathic drugs. The combination may produce dangerous reactions, allergies and have harmful side effects. Sometimes homeopathic medicines are contaminated with steroids and other dangerous chemicals. This is because steroids produce rapid symptomatic relief of fever, pain, sneezing and wheezing. They suppress the symptoms while silently exacerbating the disease and delaying the diagnosis and cure.

As a patient :

➤ Do not accept Homeopathic, Sidha or Herbal medications from a practitioner of allopathic medicine. They lack the expertise to dose correctly in that system of medicine. Treatment based on hearsay and anecdotes is not scientific.

➤ Similarly, do not accept allopathic medication from a practitioner of alternative medicine. Their expertise is elsewhere and experience is not a substitute for education and training.

➤ Interventions like magnetic therapy (provided you are not on a pacemaker), acupuncture, aroma therapy, massage, yoga, tai chi, reiki, reflexology, shiatsu, colour and crystal therapy can be used to enhance the benefit from all systems.

➤ Whenever you go to a physician take all you medical documents with you. Inform them if you are on medication from other systems of medicine.

> ➢ Choose a system of medicine that suits you best. Do not mix and match. The interactions of the medications are not known and it may be dangerous to your health.

Alternative therapy involving exercise, body manipulations, massages, meditation and lifestyle modifications are harmless. They may provide tremendous benefits as they bring the patient into contact with like minded people with similar problems providing a much needed support group.

> ➢ "Energy therapy" focuses on the harnessing energy fields from ones own body, and then redirecting it, to balance equilibrium, prevent illness and promote well-being.

> ➢ "Meditation" can be used to attain spirituality and is self directed. It can also harness and direct the body's own energy inwards to affect bodily functions and symptoms and facilitate healing. Intense concentration on a particular object or sound for a specified length of time helps to focus the mind and clears it of stress.

> ➢ Standing is one of the easiest forms of therapy to practice. It involves standing still, with the feet apart, balanced on the heels, with the knees slightly bent, arms stretched out and head held straight, with the gaze fixed steadily ahead.

> ➢ "Light healing touch" unleashes the body's own untapped healing potential by using the body's own energy fields. Charts are available showing the acupressure points to be touched. The energy unleashed harnesses health, prevents illness, accelerates healing, induces peace and promotes a feeling of well being.

> ➢ Relaxation techniques, involve progressive muscle relaxation, which starts from the head or foot and proceeds up or down. It is accompanied by deep breathing and soft soothing music. Mood elevating endorphins are released, relieving pain, reducing fatigue and stress, lowering blood pressure and inducing sleep. Good sleep itself helps to cure many illnesses and produce a relaxed feeling of well being.

> ➤ "Guided imagery" involves concentrating and visualizing a particular area that requires treatment and then curing the disease by thought, step by step.

> ➤ "Magnetic therapy" is based on the fact that the earth has a magnetic field which influences the movement of water. Since the human body is mainly composed of water, theoretically magnets can realign and balance the body's own internal electromagnetic fields. This facilitates self-healing by improving circulation, cellular oxygenation, and metabolism. Blood flow can be redirected to specific areas to reduce pain and inflammation.. Also, magnets are believed to activate electrical charges that release neurotransmitters and decrease blood pressure. They should be avoided in people fitted with pacemakers or metallic prosthetic parts.

Systems of physical exercise that focus on the mind as well as the body like yoga, Tai chi, aerobics, and the martial arts are universally beneficial irrespective of the person's age and illness. They all increase muscle tone and decrease reaction time.

Physical exercise makes the body "fighting fit," elevates mood, reduces the duration of illness and provides the ability to cope.

At times, doctors fail to realize that human beings are not just complex collections of biological matter. They live in societies, in dynamic equilibrium with the environment, friends, family and cultural beliefs. A disturbance in this balance changes the quality of their life and requires unwelcome adjustments. This may be enough to produce physical and stress related psychosomatic illnesses. Ill health cannot be treated successfully with medicine alone without tackling all the interrelated factors.

Alternative therapy externally used does provide stress reduction, rejuvenation and a feeling of control over life in today's fast paced electronically connected and wireless world.

In situations which require palliation as there is no possibility of a cure, in combination with allopathic medicine, it adds to pain relief, provides symptom control and psychosocial and spiritual support. It is combatable with prevailing cultural and ethnic practices.

The positive steps taken, helps people to overcome feelings of frustration, dissatisfaction and despair about disease processes and the quality of life.

Quackery? Perhaps, but sometimes it works.

CHAPTER 67

VITAMIN AND MINERAL SUPPLEMENTS

"Less is Bad, More is Worse"

Media publicity has highlighted the potential hazards of stress, pollution, lack of sleep, consumption of artificially fertilized and engineered crops and the new urban life style. This has resulted in health being slickly packaged and marketed as a profitable commodity. Nutritional supplements and vitamins, once prerogatives of the sick, bedridden and elderly are now considered essential.

The pharmaceutical companies vie with each other with claims, marketing gimmicks and eye-catching advertisements for irrational formulations. Advertisements prey on fears of disease, poor pregnancy outcomes, and retarded physical and mental development.

Aware of this dangerous trend, government legislation has fixed the price and the composition of vitamin and mineral formulations. This has forced manufacturers to repackage vitamins as "dietary supplements" which are not under "price control" by adding trace elements, amino acids and minerals to the original formulation. The price is higher, but the proportions of the constituents are not scientific, nor are the advantages of the additives proved.

Two favourites are "biotin" and methionine. Deficiency of biotin is rare except in those who eat raw eggs, but the compound itself is relatively harmless. Extra supplements of methionine on the other hand are harmful in the absence of a proven deficiency, if the diet is already deficient in homocysteine or folic acid, or during pregnancy.

Vitamin supplements may be purchased OTC (over the counter) or prescribed by your doctor. It pays to be knowledgeable about what is actually required and what you are about to take.

Some "high potency" vitamin supplements provide one ingredient in high concentrations and the rest in sub optimal doses. Timed release formulas cost more. They are not worth the extra expense. Each tablet may provide the requirements in sub optimal doses so that you actually need to swallow three or more doses per day to get the required concentration. If the package says "once a day" don't take it twice, you will be doing your self more harm than good. If you are taking both fortified food supplements and medication, check the total concentration of constituents as it may eventually add up to toxic doses.

Vitamin A occurs naturally as carotenoids in yellow foods. Lack of the vitamin usually does not occur in the normal state unless precipitated by malabsorption. Excess consumption is dangerous and can result in hypervitaminosis A. In children it causes symptoms similar to that of a brain tumour. Excessive consumption of carotenoids, causes a yellow discoloration of the skin. Retinoids, the precursor of vitamin A is administered as a treatment for acne. In a pregnant woman this can cause severe congenital malformations.

Vitamin D prevents rickets. Inadvertent administration of excessive doses causes hypotonia,. Irritability, vomiting, metastatic calcification, aortic valvular stenosis, and clouding of the cornea and conjunctiva.

Vitamin K is needed for clotting. Excessive administration of synthetic vitamin K can produce liver damage.

The B complex vitamins usually exhibit their deficiency a group and produce fatigue, irritability, skin changes, anaemia, burning feet, fissures angles of the mouth and a smooth red tongue. Excess vitamins are usually harmlessly excreted in the urine.

However, pregnant women given high doses of vitamin B6 (pyridoxine) to counter vomiting can produce children with B6 dependency, and convulsions.

More than 65 mg a day of iron should not be taken. Men usually do not need iron supplementation.

More than 60 mg a day of zinc may be harmful

Men and women over 50 need 1200 mg a day of calcium. More than 2500 mg should not be taken.

Amino acids are the basic building blocks of all protein and are added to dietary supplements. Deficiency in the absorption and utilization of amino acids occurs as a genetic defect. Affected individuals manifest in child hood with mental retardation or convulsions and do not survive into adult life.

Total protein deficiency due to illness or malnutrition manifests with generalized swelling of the body and changes in the hair and nails. A few milligrams of amino acid in a capsule or tonic will not help.

Iodine is provided in "iodized salt." Supplements and tonics sometimes provide additional iodine. This inadvertent intake can confound the clinical picture and make adjustments of dosage of thyroid medication difficult as the thyroid disease gets out of control.

Pregnant women require folic acid supplements. Some expensive "women's supplements" are marketed with additional herbs and amino acids. This is not needed and may actually be dangerous.

Some special rejuvenating preparations for men contain sub optimal doses of herbs whose benefit is questionable. Sometimes androgens, testosterone and other hormones are added to these herbs which may not be required and may be harmful as well. .

Who then actually needs vitamin and mineral supplements?

In most people a sensible low fat diet supplemented with fresh fruits and vegetables supplies all the nutrients vitamins and minerals needed. Supplements are required if the diet becomes inadequate as a result of premature birth, aging, pregnancy, disease, pollution, stress and food faddism.

Remember, additives and supplements can be dangerous instead of beneficial.

When profit is the driver, ethics take a back seat, and the patient is the victim.

Chapter 68

Self-Medication is Dangerous

The woman held out a plastic box and looked at me hopefully. "Doctor can you look through these tablets and see if anything can be used before prescribing something new?"

There was a hotchpotch of medicines inside. A partially open packet of a low calorie sweetener had spilled; there were dented discoloured capsules and strange malodorous brown syrup in an unlabelled bottle.

"Don't you ever finish the course prescribed?"

The lady smiled. "When I feel better I stop the tablets. If my neighbour has the same symptoms I give some to her. Sometimes I show the used strips to the medical shop salesman and buy medicines myself."

Unregulated OTC (over the counter) sales of schedule H (medications to be dispensed by prescription only) drugs are not only illegal; they may be dangerous to the recipient. Medicines ideally should be prescribed by qualified medical personnel in the correct dose for the appropriate ailment.

In children the dose is calculated based on the body weight, and not as "small child half tablet" or "older child one tablet". The doses also have to be adjusted in senior citizens, as their kidneys and liver are less efficient at metabolizing detoxifying and excreting medications.

Drug reactions can occur especially in people concurrently on other medications for chronic ailments or those who have renal or liver decompensation.

Some drugs are contraindicated below a certain age, and others during pregnancy and breast feeding.

The most misused OTC drugs are the antibiotics. Patients self medicate, either of their own accord or with the connivance of the friendly neighbourhood chemist. For a "cold" they take paracetemol, a sedating antihistamine, and an antibiotic, the favourites being ciprofloxacin, amoxycillin, tetracycline or septran.

If the infection is viral it will subside of its own accord in around three days without an antibiotic. Viral infections have to run their course, and symptomatic treatment of pain fever and fatigue is all that is required. Prophylactic administration of an antibiotic does not help in a normal individual. It may do more harm than good, as it masks the symptoms of the real illness, produces inconclusive laboratory results and delays eventual diagnosis.

If the infection is due to disease producing virulent bacteria then a single dose is only going to suppress the infection, not cure it. The bacteria temporarily stop multiplying, and once the medication has been eliminated from the patients system, the symptoms and infection return with renewed virulence.

Inappropriate and inadequate antibiotic use results in the organism being able to overcome any resistance provided by the medicine. It then begins to thrive in the presence of the antibiotic and the patient has a relapse. Meanwhile the resistant bacteria are released into the environment and contaminate the air water and soil. The medication will not work, and friends neighbours and by-standers may acquire an infection with a virulent resident organism that mysteriously does not respond to treatment.

Fear of side effects or financial constraints force the patient to buy half or less of the prescribed amount of medication. They may decide to take it only on alternate days to prevent side effects, or to take in twice a day instead of four times. All these modifications are self defeating and render the medicine useless.

Patients fear dependency on long term medication particularly that prescribed for diabetes hypertension and other chronic long-standing ailments.

To get the best results from medication

➤ Ensure that instructions are clear about why, when and how to take medication.

➤ The time taken for a medication to be completely excreted varies in different drugs. It is not dependent on "potency."

➤ To ensure patient compliance and increase medication intervals, pharmaceutical companies are trying to make long acting formulations.

➤ Medication has to be taken at the intervals prescribed.

➤ Once a day means at the same time every day, to maintain adequate consistent drug levels for all the 24 hours. It does not mean in the morning one day and in the evening the next. Twice a day means every 12 hours. Three times a day means every 8 hours. Four times a day means every 6 hours.

➤ The total number of days medication has to be taken depends on the site of infection, the type of bacteria and on the antibiotic used. Newer or more expensive does not necessarily mean stronger or better.

When you take an allopathic medication, the chemical composition, side effects and drug interactions are known studied documented and available on the internet. Unfortunately the same is not true of traditional systems of medicine. Recently warnings have appeared in medical journals about unacceptable levels of heavy metals contaminating unregulated medications in alternative systems of medicine.

For precise and successful treatment, an accurate diagnosis has to be made. Each infective episode, viral or bacterial is unique and not caused by the same organism. Treatment therefore has to be tailored to the individual and the disease. A regimen that worked last time may not succeed a second time, unless it is a recurrence of the same infection, nor is it likely to benefit friends and neighbours.

Take medication only as prescribed.

Do not self medicate.

Do not take mysterious unnamed undocumented injections and tablets.

CHAPTER 69

COSMETIC INTERVENTIONS

Looking good feeling great

Aging is inevitable universal and stressful. "Looking young and feeling good", is a 21st century mantra chanted by both men and women in today's high tech world. Sagging grey skin, unsightly spots, crow's feet, cracked lips and lines at the angles of the mouth are a dead giveaway of the passage of time. Areas constantly wrinkled develop permanent lines, especially while squinting at the computer, frowning, or rubbing an itchy nose upwards. Exposure of unprotected skin to the ultraviolet rays of sunlight, or to the dry temperature controlled atmosphere of an air-conditioned work place, produces skin with a dry dull aged appearance.

Physical appearance also now just has a price tag attached. Age or the appearance of age reduces job opportunities. This has spawned and industry where you can buy the face you want and purchase the appearance you desire. There is an epidemic of dyed hair and bleached skin affecting both sexes across the country. With these and other subtle interventions, it is possible to keep prospective employers, family members and the general public guessing.

To keep your skin looking young,

➢ Avoid exposure to sunlight by carrying an umbrella.

➢ Concentrate on smiling to avoid developing an age induced unattractive downward droop and sagging of the angles of the mouth.

➢ Apply a small amount of a mixture of oils (500ml coconut oil, 500ml of sesame oil, 100 ml of olive oil) in the evening for 10 minutes. Massage this with a firm circular motion around the eyes to prevent crow's feet, puffiness under the eyes and droopy eyelids. Stretch the neck upwards and rub on the chin and downwards to the neck.

➤ Wash this off with a herbal mixture (500 gms masoor dhal powdered with 500 gms of green gram and 100gms of Kasturi manjal). If this sounds difficult use a mild ready to use face wash (not really recommended except in emergencies).

➤ A well-balanced diet with carotenoids, antioxidants, the fat soluble vitamins A, D and E and adequate hydration help to maintain skin tone and turgur.

➤ Regular exercise, walking, jogging and yoga give the skin a healthy glow that money and makeup cannot buy.

These interventions are inexpensive and easy. However, for the brave and well heeled there are several invasive interventions to provide the "elixir for eternal youth".

A surgical "facelift" can tighten the skin and smoothen out wrinkles. At the same time the jaw line, which tends to merge with the neck as age advances can be recreated. Surgical intervention lasts, but has a prolonged recovery time. For the unfortunate there is always the risk of a devastating infection producing an aesthetically unacceptable result. If the person is prone to keloids, unsightly hyper-pigmented itchy elevations may appear along the surgery lines.

The outline of the lips can be changed and wrinkles smoothened out by using injections. A special fluid containing collagen fat silicone or botox can be used.

Collagen is an animal protein and is safer than silicone. However, allergy is a real problem and a skin test should be done before it is used. It is also very expensive, so sometimes only small quantities are used to fill the areas between wrinkles. The effects of collagen injections last 3–6 months after which they have to be repeated.

A person's fat can be harvested from one area with liposuction and injected in other required areas. This avoids allergic reactions. The fat is absorbed very slowly and therefore the procedure requires several sittings. Small quantities have to be injected each time to prevent development of a bizarre appearance.

Silicone is available in hard and soft forms and is injected into the required areas. The hard version is easier to remove should the surgical results be unsatisfactory. The soft version tends to stick to the inside of skin and nerves making it difficult to remove. If the injection was in the wrong place the skin develops an unsightly red blotchy appearance.

The popular botox injections temporarily paralyze the injected area. No wrinkles appear while smiling and crow's feet also disappear. The effect lasts for 3–6 months.

Newer procedures are on the anvil.

Thernmage thermacool is used instead of face lifts by many celebrities including Oprah Winfrey. It is a technique that uses radio frequencies to heat the collagen and smoothen out wrinkles. Each sitting lasts about an hour.

Laser techniques are being developed to remove the outer layers of the eyelid, tighten facial skin, eliminate unsightly spots and open skin pores. All of which hopefully will give the skin a youthful appearance.

Before embarking on surgical interventions

➢ Check if the doctor is a qualified plastic surgeon.
➢ Ensure that the nursing home has adequate facilities.
➢ Ask others who have had treatment what their reactions were.
➢ Look at treated people and decide if that is really what you want.

Remember appreciation of beauty, or evaluation of age, is subjective, and only in the mind of the person, and eyes of the beholder.

CHAPTER 70

CHOOSING PROPER FOOTWEAR

The boy, all of three years stepped excitedly out of the red omni, and fell flat on his face. It was not surprising, both his feet were squeezed into sandals with different designs belonging to the left foot.

"Why have you done this?" I asked.

The mother's answer was direct and to the point,

"He is always losing his right sandal. I am left with two left shoes. Do you know how expensive they are?"

That may be true, but placing the remaining left foot sandals on both feet is not the answer! The right and left soles are cut with different angulations in the factory and the wrong foot cannot be forcefully inserted into a shoe without inflicting damage. Children's feet are still growing and developing. Alignment has to be correct from the beginning to prevent lifelong pain and problems.

Our feet take a great deal of wear and tear. From the time we attain mobility (around the age of one) until we become bed-ridden they transverse thousands of kilometres.

The point is, are you going to undertake this journey in comfort or in agony?

Children do not need shoes until they start to walk confidently. Their grip on the floor is stronger if they are barefoot. Their feet need the time to grow and they need to explore and understand the textures of different flooring. Even after that, footwear should have at least a thumb's space between the toe and the end of the foot, the heel should be sturdy but not confining, the material should allow the feet to breathe. This means synthetic plastics, 'rexine' and 'sandak' should be avoided.

Socks should be made either out of pure cotton, or a 60 percent cotton-40 percent nylon/polyster/lycra mix. NOT out of pure nylon. Nylon does not allow sweat to permeate or evaporate. This leaves the foot hot sticky and damp and predisposes to fungal infection.

Shoes should be aired and socks washed after each use.

Schools add to the problem. The deciding factor about the style of footwear recommended by the school should be a combination of quality and cost. Natural material like leather or cloth should be used instead of synthetic material.

Children trend to sustain injuries either by wearing the wrong kind of shoe. Sometimes their feet are twisted and bent. They may have out grown the shoe but be forced to wear it anyway. Sometimes the shoes are too loose and large, as parents hope they will grow into it.

Schools issue "standard footwear" as part of the uniform even though the size of the child's foot varies. Schools ignore Individual variations and requirements in footwear. Instead, corporal punishment is inflicted for a failure to conform. Medical certificates or letters are ignored.

Adults sometimes torture themselves. Corns, painful calluses and throbbing soles are self-inflicted by ill-fitting, badly repaired and worn-out footwear. Part of the heel may be on the floor. The toe area may be torn necessitating a crab like gait to prevent the sandal from flying off. This ensuing faulty gait causes pain in the foot. The unstable gait may cause pain extending to the hip and knee as well.

Shoes can be replaced for a price but the feet are priceless.

Teenage girls torture their feet tottering on fashionable spikes. Sometimes, they hobble in tight footwear with asymmetrically fixed square block heels. Their balance is off-centre and every staircase or bump on the road feels like an obstacle course. They may loose their balance resulting in frequent sprains and other injuries. Resulting torn ligaments can cause lifelong instability in the joint.

Earlier, Indian homes were plastered with mud and cow dung. Soft on the feet, pliant and resilient, it made the absence of carpeting immaterial and footwear at home redundant. Times have changed. Marble and mosaic make floors granite hard. Feet are forced to navigate this flooring day after day. Fluid collects under the hard skin of the foot near the heel causing plantar fasciitis. Our barefoot housewives are unable to place their feet on the ground in the morning when they get up without an involuntary "ouch" as a shooting pain moves upwards like an electric shock.

Women should be encouraged to wear rubber slippers in the house. Worn-out parts should either be replaced promptly or the slipper abandoned as an asymmetrical sole alters the balance and produces repetitive injury.

Shoes slippers and sandals should be purchased in the evening when the feet are slightly swollen after the day's work. They should be tried in the standing position and must be comfortable when first worn. There is no question of breaking in footwear. This is a myth perpetuated by slick salesmen anxious to make a deal. Both feet should be comfortable as one foot may be fractionally larger than the other. As far as possible the material should be natural and not synthetic. The sole and heel should have firm non-slippery grip.

Proper athletic (canvas) shoes must be used for sporting activity. There should be no bare foot or slipper clad basketball!.

A lifetime of discomfort and pain can be avoided by early attention to detail.

Take care of your feet. Unlike your shoes, they are irreplaceable!.

CHAPTER 71

CRACKED AND FISSURED FEET

At the beauty competition, one of the judges kept leaning over and peering at the ground as the beautifully dressed girls paraded on the make shift cat walk.

"What are you doing?"

"Beauty extends to the feet. Anyone who does not look after their feet well does not deserve a title."

The idea was contagious, and soon all the judges were peering at the feet of the contestants.

Surprisingly, a few had dirty feet with misshapen uncut and irregular toenails. In others, constant use of tight fitting, user unfriendly, foot wear had produced cramped toes bent on each other. Some had cracked and fissured heels with dark dirt lines in the crevices.

The visual impact of expensive fashionable designer out fits was be marred by the ill- fitting footwear and fissured heels.

Our feet are visible because of our penchant for open toed back less slippers and sandals. Very few people wear closed shoes. Cracked heels, unkempt toenails and dry skin are unsightly. The crevices in-between can become filled with dirt. Contact with detergent and water then can cause infection, particularly in people who have diabetes.

All skin constantly dies, is shed and replenished. This process is automatic and carefully controlled. When the control slips, the skin becomes thick (hyperkeratosis). The soles of the feet are particularly prone to this. The thick layer of dead skin develops cracks under pressure of the body's weight. It is worse in people with obesity, dry skin, or genetic illnesses like icthyosis or psoriasis.

Unsightly corns can appear because of constant uneven pressure on the feet while standing and walking. This may be because foot wear is worn out and has cracked soles. Gait automatically subconsciously adjusts to reduce pain. Lurching and slightly off-centre movement not only produces corns, but eventually leads to knee and hip problems.

Sometimes feet are squeezed into stylish foot wear that is too tight or too small. Toes get pushed together. Over a long time they can become misshapen and misaligned. If the heel of the foot sticks out at the back the hard sole of the slipper cuts into and it develops pain. If footwear is too loose, it flops around providing no support and interfering with balance. It may suddenly fly off at inconvenient moments especially while trying to move fast.

Traditionally, foot wear is not used inside Indian homes. That was fine as long as bathing and washing places were outside, and the water drained away or sank rapidly into the absorbent earth. Now, floors are hard and non-absorbent. Consequently, feet may be immersed in detergent containing water and they develop cracks. This makes women more prone to develop cracked feet than men.

Initially, if the cracks are too deep and tedious to remove, beauty parlours have professionals, who will scrub the excess skin off with ardour. Do not allow them to attack your feet with blades and scissors to cut off thickened or excess skin. This short cut is dangerous, as any break in the deeper layers of intact skin may allow infection to occur.

Many creams and lotions are advertised in the media for cracked feet. They are expensive and inefficient.

- ➤ At home, to maintain smooth heels,
- ➤ Soak the feet for 10 mins once a week in a basin of warm water to which a teaspoon of liquid soap and a tablespoon of rock salt has been added.
- ➤ Then clean the soles of the feet especially at the heel with a plastic brush.
- ➤ Next, scrub the heels with a foot scrubber, available in supermarkets. Apply non greasy body oil to the feet and heels every night.

Soaking also softens the nails and they can be easily and safely cut at the same time, using a nail cutter. After cutting the nails file them carefully. Take care to see that the skin on the sides of the nail is not cut. That can cause a painful infection and swelling.

Give yourself a foot massage with oil once a week. It keeps the skin healthy and reduces mental stress.

If here are any corns treat them as they start to develop, not after they are hard painful. Commercial corn caps are available and effective if they are used precisely as instructed on the leaflet.

Care of the feet must become a regular habit. If it is physically difficult to bend down, observe your feet and care for them, it is time to loose the extra flab around your middle.

Some multinational companies have dress codes in which it is clearly stated that women have to have pedicured feet! Failure to conform can result in loss of the job.

Care for your feet well. They are the ornamental pedestals on which you undertake your journey through life.

CHAPTER 72

TACKLING ANIMAL BITES

The four year old boy was screaming at the top of his voice as he clutched his bleeding scalp, his mother was ineffectively flapping her arms around, and his grandmother had quietly fainted. They had been on an innocuous enough family expedition, a picnic to a forest area, where he had sustained an unprovoked wild monkey bite. Fortunately for him, the dramatic nature of the incident ensured that the family rushed for medical aid.

Many others are not as lucky. They come into casual contact with wild animals, strays, domesticated animals or pets, and are unaware that it is not just penetrative injury, but also cuts, scratches or even licks on abraded or damaged mucosal surfaces and skin, which can give the rabies virus a point of entry. Rabies is a dangerous and fatal disease. Monkeys, along with wolves, foxes, mongooses, bats, cats and dogs carry the rabies virus.

Transmission of rabies from one human to another does not occur from bites or contamination with saliva. It has only been documented internationally in seven cases of corneal transplantation. In India, there are between 40,000 to 70,000 cases of rabies reported a year. The exact incidence is not known, as the incubation period varies from days to months. The initial contact with animal may not be remembered, as it was trivial, and not significant enough to be taken seriously.

Even if the animal is a pet, the immunizations given to it may not be adequate or up to date. Booster doses may have been missed or forgotten. Besides, immunized cats and dogs kept as pets can be asymptomatic carriers of rabies. They can then transmit the disease to their unsuspecting owners and others.

The number of cases of rabies caused by injuries inflicted by cats is greater that that caused the more publicized dog bites in the USA.

Why should this be so?

It is difficult to confine cats, even when they are pampered pets. They escape, wander free and sustain injuries in fights with other canines. There is a reservoir of infection in the forests in wild animals, from which infection feasible, if the animal is a stray or has run back to the forest.

Irrespective, the treatment does not change. The wound has to be cleaned well with a 20 percent soap solution. This is veridical, and reduces the load of viruses in the wound. Iodine solution should then be used either tincture iodine or as commercially available povidone iodine solution. Suturing should be avoided as that produces a closed environment allows further multiplication of the viruses.

Immunoglobulins commercially available on prescription from medical shops, should be infiltrated by a doctor around the wound, and post exposure prophylaxis (after the bite treatment) started with anti-rabies vaccine. Prior to the advent of the human diploid cell and other newer vaccines, this involved injection of the vaccine in the abdomen around the navel. The old regimen had many side effects, of which pain was the least sinister and most tolerable!

A number of companies market the newer vaccines. They are freely available. The dosage schedule is printed on the package insert and should be meticulously followed. Post-exposure prophylaxis is usually given on days 0,3,5,7,14 and 28. The site of injection is important. Injections should be administered in the shoulder intramuscularly and not the buttocks. This is because the high fat content in the buttocks interferes with adequate antibody production.

In addition, bites require tetanus prophylaxis, and antibiotic cover against aerobic and anaerobic bacteria which may infect the wound from the teeth of the animal.

Pre-exposure prophylaxis (before the bite) consists of three injections given on days 0,7,28 with a booster every 5 years. It should be offered to all owners of pet dogs or cats, veterinary surgeons, laboratory workers, and travellers especially if they are going to pass through endemic areas here appropriate treatment for animal bites may not be readily available.

With awareness, pre exposure prophylaxis and knowledge the fear associated with animal bites can be greatly reduced.

CHAPTER 73

RESUSCITATION

ABC and CPR-- Saving Lives

The anecdotal ancient "God of death" found in most ancient cultures comes to claim the soul when your time on earth is up. Even rationalists begin to lend credence to this theory when people of all ages, infants, children, adolescents and young adults suddenly "keel over and drop dead", for no obvious reason at all. Sometimes, they die in their sleep and do not wake up.

Death occurs when the brain stops functioning. Sudden death occurs in the absence of recognized pre-existing illness if the blood supply to the brain is insufficient. Life giving oxygen is supplied to the brain through blood vessel pipelines by the pumping of the heart. This pump can fail as a result of a block in the blood vessels or an internal electrical malfunction of the heart muscles.

The oxygen breathed in may not reach the blood due to an obstruction in the airways or a breakdown of the lung function. The blood vessels themselves may collapse as a result of over whelming infection or uncontrolled hypertension.

If there is sudden unexpected collapse or death, the presence of mind and prompt action of by-stander with knowledge of CPR (cardio- pulmonary resuscitation), can save lives.

CPR should be taught in high schools and colleges. Medical personnel can be invited to give demonstrations and lectures. CPR techniques, to circulate blood and oxygen through the body, can be performed manually without any machines. This keeps the brain alive. If it is successfully initiated within 4 minutes, the survival rate is 40%. However, the survival rate drops to 10% if there is a delay of 8 minutes.

15 % of people will have the opportunity to perform CPR at sometime in their lives. If they do not know the techniques, they will have to watch helplessly as someone's life ebbs away.

Procedure

If a person has collapses suddenly, first loosen any constricting clothing. Then administer a thump to the front of the chest. If this is unsuccessful proceed to CPR.

Basic resuscitation can be remembered as ABC.

A stands for airway and this has to be clear. If it is blocked with blood, mucous, a foreign body (bones nuts) or water, air cannot enter.

- ➤ Perform the Heimlich manoeuvre. This may have to be repeated a few times. (Explained in the next chapter).
- ➤ Place the person on his back on a firm surface
- ➤ Extend the neck gently back wards (chin lift) and extend the head (head lift). This is the position one naturally assumes when smelling a strange odour.
- ➤ Do not remove dentures as they provide a firm support for the jaw.
- ➤ Once the airway is clear, proceed to step 2.

B stands for breathing.

Listen and look for breathing by placing your cheek close to the person's mouth and watching for the rise and fall of the abdomen.

If the person is not breathing

- ➤ Pinch the victim's nostrils firmly
- ➤ Place your mouth over the victim's mouth
- ➤ Blow air in forcefully at the rate of 1 breath per second.

The same technique can be performed safely in infants and children. Expired air provides enough oxygen for survival.

If the mouth is full of vomited material or blood in then a rescuer may feel reluctant to administer mouth to mouth resuscitation. In such cases administering chest compressions alone may help and is better than masterly inactivity.

C stands for circulation

Circulatory collapse can be confirmed by feeling for the carotid pulse in the angle of the jaw. It is located on both sides 2 cms below the angle of the jaw in front of the big neck muscle called the sternocleidomastoid. If the carotid pulse is not felt, or you are doubtful about its location, do not waste more than 10 seconds.

Proceed with cardiac resuscitation.

- ➤ Place the heel of one hand over the lower half of the sternum.
- ➤ Place the heel of the second hand on top of the first .
- ➤ Keep the arms straight.
- ➤ Rhythmically depress the sternum 2–5cms at the rate of 100 compressions per min.
- ➤ In children use the thumbs one on top of the other and press down only 1–2 cms.

It is easier if two people work in tandem, with 15 chest compressions to 2 breaths (15:2) ratio. If resuscitating alone, stop chest compressions while breathing into the persons mouth.

Chest compressions do not directly massage the heart. The pressure is transmitted through the closed chest to the heart, which is naturally fitted with valves that ensure forward circulation from the heart to the rest of the body.

Oriental culture dictates that if you save someone's life, your souls are intertwined and they are indebted to you forever. The God of death has decided to by pass them and give them a second lease of life on borrowed time attached to another soul.

What can be more satisfactory?

CHAPTER 74

CHOKING

Ever Heard of Dr. Henry Heimlich?

Elizabeth Taylor would have died choking on a chicken bone if the waiter in the restaurant had not paid attention when the Heimlich manoeuvre was taught in his first aid class. He not only knew who Heimlich was, but performed his manoeuvre with sufficient expertise to dislodge the bone and save her life.

Choking is a great social equalizer. It cuts across boundaries and affects all kinds of people. The famous, unknown, young, old, rich or poor all choke unexpectedly on food particles, coins, seeds and nuts. Many die before they received medical aid.

Much of this has changed after the Heimlich manoeuvre was widely demonstrated in the media, scientifically taught, and popularized as a first aid measure.

Dr. Heimlich actually discovered that compression of the abdomen below the level of the rib cage pushes air forcefully out of the lungs dislodging any foreign body causing an obstruction to breathing, thus saving lives.

Suspect that a person's airway is blocked if:

A conscious victim cannot breathe, cough or speak to ask for help.

- The person's face turns blue.
- The person desperately grabs at his or her throat.
- The person has a weak cough, breathing is difficult.
- A high-pitched noise is produced with each breath..

After a few frantic nerve wracking minutes, they may change in colour and fall down unconscious. Delay in action at this point can lead to death.

An unconscious person is non-responsive. Do not wait for assistance to arrive as it may be too late. It is better to start to perform the manoeuvre before trying to verify if there is a heart beat or pulse. Anyone can perform the Heimlich manoeuvre.

You may save a life!

The basic manoeuvre works well in a conscious person even though they are panic stricken, as they may cooperate to some extent.

- Wrap your arms around the victim's waist from behind.
- Make a fist with your hand and place it against the victim's upper abdomen, just below the ribcage but above the umbilicus. Place the thumb closest to the person's body
- Place your other hand on top of the first one.
- Grasp your fist with your other hand and press into your upper abdomen with quick upward thrusts.
- Repeat until object is expelled.

Excessive force is not required. It may fracture the bones of chest and rib cage and damage internal organs. The sharp jerks may also cause vomiting. If this occurs turn the head to one side. Aspiration of the vomited material may lead to further choking and secondary infection, making the cure almost as bad as the disease.

If a person is lying on the floor, unconscious, or it is not possible to reach all the way around, (obesity or pregnancy) do not slap them on the back or lift their feet as this may worsen the problem.

Instead,

- Position the person on the back face up.
- Kneel astride (straddle) on the hips
- Place the fist under the sternum
- Thrust in the same way as above

In infants, care must be taken to place them flat on a firm surface before gently performing the same procedure, using the fingers instead of the fists.

A person who was drowning and was pulled out of the water and needs to have the water removed from the lungs first. Air cannot enter unless water leaves. They need to be placed on hard ground and turned to one side as the manoeuvre is performed. This is to help water drain out of the lungs and prevent aspiration of stomach contents.

If the person was choking (not drowning) on fluids then this manoeuvre performed in an upright position will expel fluids.

If choking or an acute asthma attack occurs when alone, do not panic. This manoeuvre can be done alone by leaning over a table edge, chair, railing or bed post and pressing the upper abdomen against the edge with sudden movements to produce a quick upward thrust..

This manoeuvre may have to be repeated several times to be successful. Thumping the person on the back or holding them upside down is not beneficial. It may actually be harmful.

Calm composure and presence of mind ensures success.

Sometimes the manoeuvre has to be followed by Cardio-Pulmonary Resuscitation or CPR. A person who has choked needs to be evaluated by a doctor as soon as possible.

Children are particularly susceptible to aspiration and choking.

- ➤ Do not feed children nuts or give them coins.
- ➤ Eat small mouthfuls chewing well.
- ➤ Concentrate and do one thing at a time. Multitasking is efficient, but it can be dangerous if it involves eating and talking at the same time.

Choking is dangerous. Prevention is safer than a cure.

Thank you Dr. Henry Heimlick!

CHAPTER 75

FIRST AID

Look in the First Aid Box

Calamity strikes and medical emergencies occur; when you are alone, in the middle of the night, when no doctors, neighbours or relatives can be summoned. A little sound knowledge about first aid, and a box in which you can rummage for remedies may go a long way towards saving lives.

The box should be kept in an accessible place out of the reach of children. It should contain:

- a pair of scissors,
- a scribbling pad and pen,
- a torch (that works),
- copies of any insurance or hospital number cards,
- a gauze bandage roll,
- a roll of cotton ,
- a few band aids,
- a tube of pain relieving ointment,
- an antiseptic ointment like povidone-iodine,
- an antibiotic ointment (bacitracin, polymixcin),
- eye drops, nose drops and analgesic ear drops.
- medications that can be stored are tablets of aspirin, paracetemol (adult and kid), an antispasmodic, and anti histamines like chlorpheniramine maleate (Avil) and diphendydramine (Benedryl), and an antacid liquid.

Chest pain causes panic in the person and bystanders with visions of sudden death. In a heart attack, remember, the pain is present for

15 minutes or longer. It radiates up the neck, down the arm, moves to the back and is associated with sweating, fainting and pallor. Medical help is urgently needed. However, before proceeding to the hospital, administer a tablet of aspirin (325mg). Aspirin has saved innumerable lives when administered in this fashion.

Toothaches are agonizing and tend to start in the middle the night. It is usually due to tooth decay. Temporarily sucking on an ice cube may help. Also, take a pain killer like aspirin paracetemol or celecoxib and then contact a dentist as soon as possible. Do not apply medication directly on the affected tooth.

Electrical short circuits, fires and shocks are very common. Substandard old wiring, moisture, or uninsulated exposed wires are dangerous. Exposed plug points in houses should be closed with plastic "plug stoppers." If some one is in contact with live electricity, always run and switch off the mains first. Do not touch a person in contact with a live electrical current without using a non conductive material such as a wooden spoon or plastic stick. Never touch a wire barefoot. Although the actual burn caused by electricity can appear small, the damage can extend deep into the body. It can cause the heart to stop beating. Violent jerking can cause dislocations and fractures.

Burns and scalds are very common. If a person is on fire do not let them run. Roll them on the ground or wrap them in a heavy sheet. This cuts off the air supply and helps to smother the fire.

If there is a burn, immediately hold the area under cool water or apply a cold compress. Directly placing ice on the burnt area is not advisable as can cause frost bite. If there is a blister wipe the area over the blister with a solution of povidone –iodine to sterilize it. Then poke it in 3 areas to release the fluid inside, keeping the overlying skin intact. This makes the skin collapse on the blister and the area is no longer raw. Then apply an antibiotic ointment and cover it with a gauze bandage which lets in air.

Fainting is usually harmless. It is due to a temporary insufficiency in the blood supply to the brain. By elevating the legs above the head, the venous return is increased rectifying this problem. Position the person on their back. Elevate the legs above the head. If the person is in the sitting position, place the head between the knees.

Any substance, natural or artificial can precipitate an allergic attack; pollen, chemicals in the air, dust, latex from gloves or shoes, or additives and colouring agents in the food. There may be signs of itching; the throat may swell, with redness and swelling of the lips and difficulty in breathing. Mild reactions can be treated with oral tablets of an antihistamine like chlorpheniramine (Avil) or diphenhydramine (Bendryl). Difficulty in breathing or swelling of the throat is an emergency. The person should be rushed to a hospital.

If an insect has entered the ear, place the ear against a bright light. The insect may fly out. Otherwise, pour a little paraffin oil or baby oil into the ear. The insect will float up. Do not attempt to pry the insect loose with an ear bud as you may damage the ear.

Nose block is very uncomfortable. With the head tilted back, place nose drops in each nostril and then take a steam inhalation. This will clear up an allergic block or one due to a cold. If there is a foreign body try to blow out gently. Close the opposite nostril and try. Do not suck in as it will move the object upwards.

Bleeding from the nose can usually be stopped by using decongescent nose drops and then pinching the nostrils together. If it occurs frequently, or is associated with easy bruising and bleeding from other sites it needs to be evaluated.

If the eye is inured by a blunt object, bleeding around the eye causes discolouration around the eye (black eye). This is usually not serious. It will subside spontaneously with a cold compress. Bilateral black eyes may to be due to head injury and are a dangerous sign.

A foreign body in the eye can cause damage to the cornea. There is usually a very specific uncomfortable sensation of grittiness. Do not rub the eye. Immediately wash the eye with running water and apply antibiotic eye drops.

If there is bleeding from any area apply pressure over the site to reduce the bleeding and proceed for help.

Be prepared and knowledgeable, it may save lives.